Here's wha

If You Loved Yourself, What Would You Do Now?

"I love this book more than I have words for. It is so important and so beautifully articulated, and I am SO thrilled someone in the world has said these things out loud so that other people in the world (like me) can heal themselves. You're a gifted writer and communicator. I'm so thrilled for you, and for me who gets to read it and learn some super important and life-changing things."

"This book has introduced a simple but profound concept into my life, one that I now refer to daily. Eilat's voice is practical, down-to-earth and relatable, and reading the book feels as easy and inspiring as having a chat with a loving friend. You know you're on-board when you find yourself rushing to the 'Parenting' chapter in a moment of conflict over breakfast cereal with your 6 year old, observing your spending habits to uncover your self-love values and choosing your dinner based on self-love rather than calories ... Eilat's acute observations about human behavior illuminate what's really going on—the happy result is a release from guilt and negativity, and a move closer to joy. The message is relevant in different ways to everyone in my life."

"Thank you for writing this book. I was not only moved by the exercises and content, but also challenged in the most gentle, loving way. And the ripple of the book has continued even when I stopped reading. I have just finished reading the Money chapter. I'm on the plane, I am sitting here above the clouds as the sun sets and the final line, 'If I loved myself, how would I create the feeling of wealth for myself in this moment?' has me in tears of wealthy gratitude. You have a way of lifting veils, of shifting perspectives, of connecting mind, body and soul. I have found myself more in tune with people since reading the book and the refrain, 'if you loved yourself what would you choose to do now?' rolls off my tongue. It has been gently embedded into my psyche like a refrain in a song. So your book ripples on, long past reading, as I'm sure is your intention."

"I'm using this tool all day. Last night when I was tempted to have a second plate of food even though I was full, it was 'If you loved yourself, what would you choose right now?' And then it helped me from feeling terribly guilty about not attending a school meeting because I was utterly exhausted. What I would choose if I loved myself was to stay at home with my family and eat a plate of nourishing food and be still. So that's what I did. I had to remind myself a few times before the discomfort went away but it really, really worked :-)"

"I think Parenting is one of my very best chapters. In those crazy, chaotic, irrational parenting moments, my phrase was always 'design flaw'. It is a design flaw that kids are most demanding and out of control when both you and they are tired, etc. That chapter has expanded my paradigm to include the greater teaching those moments provide. And I feel quite normal now. And I love your sense of humor here."

"Eilat, the way you write wreathes the reader in love. What I mean is this is not just a theoretical instruction about love, but actually an experience of the thing. And I love your personal sharing. We readers love to get personal with the writer."

"Imagine finding a simple technique that can apply to all areas of 'stuckness' in your life, and that reacquaints you with the most important person in your life: You. The Love question does that and more by lovingly reconnecting you with your Truth, and providing gentle guidance in decisions big and small. If everyone did this, it would change the world."

Eilat Aviram

IF YOU LOVED YOURSELF
WHAT WOULD YOU DO NOW?

In Your Life

First edition 2019

Copyright © 2019 Eilat Aviram

www.eilataviram.com

ISBN 9781082334641

Front cover design by Gill Attwood

Illustration © by Eilat Aviram

Back cover design by Neil Bester

Editor Nicola Rijsdijk

Author photograph by Janine Kuschke Van Der Tuin

Design by Tarryn George

Printed in South Africa by Digital Action (Pty) Ltd

All rights reserved

The moral right of the author has been asserted

No part of this publication may be reproduced, distributed, or transmitted in any form or by any means, including photocopying, recording, or other electronic or mechanical methods, without the prior written permission of the author, except in the case of brief quotations embodied in critical reviews and certain other non-commercial uses permitted by copyright law.

The advice and strategies found within may not be suitable for every situation. This work is sold with the understanding that neither the author nor the publisher are held responsible for the results accrued from the advice in this book.

Contents

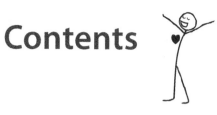

Part One: Discover the surprisingly easy Love question

1: Your only task is to live as yourself 15
2: What the Love question reveals and why 27
3: How to use the Love question 49

Part Two: You can master self-love everywhere in your life

4: If I loved myself in my Work.. 69
5: If I loved myself in my Body and Health 101
6: If I loved myself in my Food 133
7: If I loved myself in my Money.. 155
8: If I loved myself in my Sex 183
9: If I loved myself in my Parenting 205

Conclusion 243

Part Three: Resources for groups and communities

Downloadable guidelines for how to read this as a group 250

Downloadable guidelines for how to bring this concept of loving yourself and listening to your Truth into your existing community (organization, church, school)......................... 250

List of exercises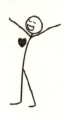

What the Love question reveals and why

Identifying your need 33
Active self-love 35
How to feel your feelings.. 37
How to make a decision in the midst of fear 43

How to use the Love question

Listening to your heart Truth 54
How does a heart answer feel? 54

If I loved myself in my Work

Ask yourself the Love question daily... 72

If I loved myself in my Body and Health

Cracking the code of your symptoms 117
How to feel joy in your body 127
How do I love my body? 129
Body map 130
How to communicate with your body 131

If I loved myself in my Food

What do I feel like eating? 143
Make love to your food (a mindfulness exercise) 145
How to love yourself through a craving 151

If I loved myself in my Money

What are your rating scales? 160
Thought-provoking questions to ask about your spending 179

If I loved myself in my Sex

A conversation with your penis or vagina 188
Fight off nothing 199

If I loved myself in my Parenting

Why does this trigger me? 212
The sweetness of loving 228

Welcome to your increased wellbeing!

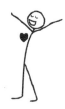

How to use this book

This book is a multimedia experience. Each chapter begins with a short meditation video to help you set an intention. There are links throughout the book to downloadable checklists and chapter summaries. All these resources are free. You can put these on your wall or fridge to support you in making self-loving choices.

You'll be asked to sign in with your email the first time you click a link and after that you'll have unlimited access to all the resources. Alternatively, access them by signing in to the member section on the website www.ifilovedmyself.com.

And remember you can use the magical technique I describe in the video on the back cover. Think of a question about yourself or your life. It can be anything – big or small. When you have the question clearly in your mind, open the book on a random page and let your eyes fall on any sentence or phrase and see how that might answer your question.

Other supportive resources:

Look for the workbook of this book that actively supports you in making the changes you want. It can really support a group working through this book together. Stickers, mugs and fridge magnets are also available to help you remember to ask the Love question in your daily life and make the changes you long for, and you can visit my website to find out how to work with me in person.

There are two books in the *If You Loved Yourself, What Would You Do Now?* series: "In Your Life" and "In Your Self". Each book offers tools to love yourself in different life areas and they are equally important; "In Your Life" explains the tool in depth and demonstrates how to use it. It covers loving yourself in your work, food, body and health, money, sex and parenting. "In Your Self" teaches how to love yourself in your thoughts and feelings, relationships, saying no, being and saying yes to life. It also looks more deeply into what love is and how to love yourself in difficult times—including trauma and shame. The two books essentially work together and it's a good idea to read both.

If at any point of reading this book you feel uncertain, just ask yourself,

"If I loved myself, what would I choose to do now?"

If you have questions, you can contact me at **www.ifilovedmyself.com**

I've used stories from my therapy room to demonstrate what it looks like to learn to love yourself. Names and details have been changed to protect people's privacy, but where the stories are recognisable I've received permission from my clients to share them. Each person has said that they're happy to offer their story in the hope that readers will gain from hearing about their experiences.

And now, a warning:

Reading this book will cause a rapid increase in self-love—almost without your realizing it—whether you're a beginner at this loving-yourself thing or already advanced.

PART ONE

DISCOVER THE SURPRISINGLY EASY LOVE QUESTION

Chapter 1

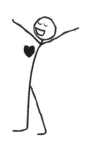

Your only task is to live as yourself

When we follow the herd we get further and further from ourselves. When we don't ask what WE want, we remove ourselves from our joy. We move ourselves away from our wholeness, from our freedom, our purpose. The things we choose to do when we love ourselves tend to be simple. We think it's going to be big and dramatic but usually the things that make us truly happy, our inner truth, is simple living and being.
Aisha Salem

Your life purpose is to be exactly who you are

Arnan sits upright on the soft couch opposite me in my psychotherapy practice, and shyly reveals his plans. His face is beaming and his energy is joyous, yet he's also nervous and I can see why. By sharing his plans, he's exposing himself, showing me his real inner being, making himself vulnerable to my opinions and reactions. These are not standard-issue hopes and dreams. They're unusual, unconventional and a little daring. His plans flout society's expectation that a young man should 'get a proper job and earn an income'.

Arnan plans to travel and explore, while working online and consulting long-distance. He wants to sail and have new experiences and flow with life. To just be. There are no office hours in these plans: just a lot of trust in himself and in life.

This is no small thing for Arnan. I've known him for several years, and I know how hard he's had to work to shake off the limitations that have been imposed on him by his family and society since childhood. I clearly remember the first number of times we met. He was confused and depressed, with thoughts of suicide, plagued by issues of health and chronic fatigue, and carrying guilt and shame about himself. He was uncertain about how he was supposed to be in the world and would desperately try to please people, constantly watching them for cues to how he should act in each moment.

At the beginning of our time together, when we talked about his Self or I asked him, "What feels right for you in this situation?" he'd look at me with confusion and panic because he didn't know what I meant. Later, when he understood the question, it frightened him more because his whole life he'd tried to suppress the 'real' him. Who he naturally was had exasperated and created stress for his parents. They like order and control, whereas he thrives in chaos, movement and change. A bright, energetic, innovative boy who always loved color and design, he was a born leader and yet, even as he was very successful in school, tertiary studies and later work, he felt anxious and purposeless and became less and less confident in himself. He wasn't listening to his Inner Truth, you see, and that will sink any spirit—even one as bright and passionate as his.

Today he sits in front of me comfortable in himself, consistently and vibrantly healthy, abundant in energy, excited about his life and purpose—such a remarkable difference. Yet I observe within myself the standard reactions to his non-standard plans and visions: *But isn't this quite irresponsible?* a stuffed-shirt part of my mind asks. *The poor boy is delusional. How does he expect to earn enough money? Traveling costs a lot. This will never work.*

I smile as these doubts come up in me and focus on him, sitting there on my couch, vibrating with joy.

Why can't he do it? I ask myself right back. *I've often seen how amazing and unpredictable life is. If he can visualize it, then it's possible. Only he can see his path and if he feels such joy about it, then it's right for him. If he doesn't do this, what will he do? For Arnan, anything else would be a compromise. And if this does work—and if it works magnificently—he'll have shown us all what can be done outside of our usual frame of reference.*

The world doesn't need more stuffed shirts. Things are changing so fast—we need people who can do things differently in a way that matches the new world order. Why should he be anything but himself?

He is here to live as himself. Anything else makes no sense at all.

This is it. This is my point and what I hope this book will give you:

You are here to live as yourself. That is your life's purpose. Anything else makes no sense at all.

You are the gift you have to give to the world. Just you, as you are—the unique combination of thoughts, behaviors, intentions, hopes, feelings and experiences that is you. It absolutely serves you better—serves all of us better—if you listen to yourself and allow yourself to simply be you. If you try to live as anyone other than yourself, we all lose out.

Like Arnan, most of us were trained to please others, to conform to what's expected and to follow what various authorities say is 'good for us'. The problem is that living according to other people's rules and ideas is more convenient for them but it doesn't meet our deeper needs and so it rarely leaves us feeling very good. Listening to other people guides us away from listening to ourselves—which is madness, because we are the sole experts on ourselves.

Why do I say you are the sole expert on yourself?

Only you can really see your own path.

Only you can know what makes *you* truly feel good—both in the tiny daily things you do and the bigger life choices you make. Other people can think they know what's best for you, but they're not living your life inside your body and mind, and so they don't have all the necessary information.

We each have our own piece of a larger puzzle to figure out—and that piece is our own life and our own Self. If we strive to copy our neighbor, nobody will ever see the bigger picture because our piece will be missing. Our singular task in life—the way we can best be of service to ourselves, our loved ones and the world—is to try to master our own part of the puzzle.

But how do we do this? Where can we start? It's easier than you think. You already have everything you need, and there's a question that can guide you every step of the way:

If I loved myself, what would I choose to do now?

That's what the rest of this book is about.

Lack of love is very bad for you

As I prepared to write this book I asked, *What do people need to know about this topic? If someone was sitting with me, what kind of questions would they have?*

I realized the first thing I'd need to do is explain what it means to love yourself. The second thing would be to motivate for why somebody should. Reflecting on this, I felt sad that *any* of us would need self-love explained and encouraged—never mind most of us! It's bizarre to have to explain why we should love ourselves. In an ideal world, we just would.

Studies on children who have not been sufficiently loved are unanimous in their conclusion: a lack of love is bad for us human beings. It's as fundamental to our optimal development as nutritious food. Children who aren't loved in the ways they need are often delayed or distorted in certain abilities and behaviors.

What is rarely pointed out is that this 'nutritional' need for love does not disappear when we become adults. For some odd reason, we seem to think that adults need less love for growth than children. This is simply not true. It's quite obvious, for example, that nutritional needs differ between youngsters and oldsters, but adults still need good food for optimal development and well-being, right? And yet as adults we often disregard our real needs—for both physical and emotional 'nutrition'.

In Part Two of this book, I've included chapters on food, health and in "In Your Self" there's a chapter on thoughts and feelings because these are all completely connected with how we love ourselves—or don't.

How we meet or ignore our needs is how we love ourselves.

Throughout this book I share powerful and intimate stories from my clients and my own life experiences as we all learn how to meet our needs. As you read on, you'll see that in every area of our lives—in disciplining our children, feeding our bodies or nourishing our souls—we need to *first* attend to love and connection. Everything else comes after.

First love, everything else after.

You already know how to do this

When was the last time you felt loved? Stop reading for a moment and really think about it. Really *filled* with love—that puffy-chested, happy, energizing, content, soft, glowing feeling?

I hope it was recently. But even if it was years ago, or never, you can get to feel it soon. Did you know that it's possible to live in that feeling all the time? There are so many things in our lives that can bring us that feeling: our own self-love, nature, good books, friends, music, children, a partner, sex, spirituality, exercising, creating ... Yet strangely, for a species that has so many ways to access this wonderful, health-inducing sensation we call love, we don't let ourselves feel it very often.

Love is incredibly good for us physically, emotionally, mentally and spiritually.

Love is actually our most natural state of being.

Think of a calm baby and how he's just open-hearted to everything he sees. Until we're trained out of our inherent behavior (which most of us are), everything we see is a wonder and everyone is welcomed with a gummy smile. A baby doesn't need to read a book on how and why to love himself: he simply doesn't know any other way to be. It's only after we've had experiences that don't affirm us—from tiny things like our mother not adequately attending to one of our needs to big things such as abuse—that we learn to be more guarded towards others, to the world and to ourselves. It's not our natural state though. We have to be *taught* to cut off from loving everything about ourselves.

You already know everything you need to about how to love yourself. You were born with that knowledge. With this book, I hope to simply trigger your memory of how to be in your inherent and natural state of self-love.

Be the source of your own love.

At some point in life many of us seem to shift from knowing love and being love to thinking that other people are responsible for giving us love. This shift only happens if we disconnect from knowing that *we* are the source of love. When you are the source of your own love, it won't occur to you to look outside of yourself to get that love because you will feel and know it all the time. Loving others and receiving love from them will just be a fun addition to how you always feel.

What do you want?

Many of us walk around accepting life as 'good enough'. This isn't a problem if 'good enough' leaves you the mental space to do your art in the evenings, or if your 'good enough' health is a great improvement on what it was before. If you are feeling elated, good and happy about where you are and what you have, keep doing what you're doing—this book will bolster your continuing joy. If, however, you're feeling disappointed with your lot, if you feel numb, disheartened or cheated by your good-enough (or completely awful) job, good-enough relationship, good-enough health and you're telling yourself, *This is just how life is, so I should grow up and stop daydreaming*, then I have very good news for you.

The feeling that your life is not quite as you'd hoped it would be, or that there's something missing, is a call from your heart to please stop and listen. Your Truth is trying to contact you.

This book offers a way to help you hear what your Truth is saying to you. We each have a 'knowing' inside ourselves, and if you feel bland or disappointed about your life in any way, it means you're not fully listening to yours—you have important needs that are currently not being met.

To learn what Truth is for you, ask the question, "If I loved myself, what would I choose to do now"? or ask, "What do I really need?" Ask this about every situation in your life that you feel less than delighted about. Then listen, speak, write, meditate, journal, travel your inner terrain ... and follow your own guidance.

No one can know Truth for anyone else. If you want to find *your* joy, you can only do so by following your inner knowing of what you deeply need and taking steps to meet those needs.

When we ask ourselves the Love question, the answer that emerges may sound totally unrealistic at first. Your response might be, *What? How can I change my career, go traveling, apply for the promotion, become an artist, end my marriage, make time for meditation ...?!*

Don't worry about making huge changes right away.

Mountains are not climbed in one or two leaps. There are many, many steps to get to the top, and if it's a big mountain, it takes more steps. Also, right now you may *think* you need to climb the whole mountain, but often as you start to make small changes, the big things shift in unexpected and surprisingly satisfying ways. Whatever life-mountain faces you, the Love question will guide you to the ideal small steps to climb it.

What does the Love question do? It directs us to the exact point where we are currently overriding our Truth or compromising ourselves in some way. All the answers you get from your Truth will be right—and realistic—for you. Bigger Truths will be offered to you already broken down into smaller manageable portions. When I say step-by-step guidance, I really mean it. Try it and see. Chapter 3 will explain how.

But why don't we just follow our Truth? It has to do with our brains. Let me explain.

Why we fear change

Fear of change often prevents us from making decisions, even when we see they could be better for us. As a species we tend to fear the unknown because the human brain is designed to avoid new things that may threaten our survival. Our brain sends out all sorts of warnings—in the form of chemicals, hormones and proteins—to stop us from making big changes with unknown outcomes (more on that in "In Your Self"). But little steps, the brain handles those better. Little steps are the best way to make big changes.

You want a happier life? Start to make your choices from a place of really listening to and respecting yourself.

Ask, *"If I loved myself, what would I choose to do now?"*

- at the dinner table when the same old argument starts with your partner
- when your boss talks to you a certain way
- when you dress in the morning
- when your partner or date wants to have sex
- when someone asks you for something ...

Moment by moment, choice by choice, you build your life. You've built your current life with the choices you've made at each decision point. What future life are you building for yourself with your choices right now?

Making the same choices you've always made will perpetuate the life you have now. Making new choices based on honoring your needs even better will create the life you're dreaming of. Pretty simple, right?

If you loved yourself, what would you choose to do now?

Are you worth loving?

Any time we do something that makes us feel bad later, it's because we didn't love ourselves in the moment we chose to do it. Not loving yourself is both the cause and the effect.

If you know something gives you a tummy ache but you keep doing it and you keep getting tummy aches, is that really a surprise? "How can I stop getting tummy aches?" you want to know. The common-sense reply is: "Stop doing the thing that causes tummy aches."

What does common sense have to say when you ask, "How can I stop feeling bad?" It says, "Stop doing things that make you feel bad and start doing things that make you feel good." In other words:

LOVE YOURSELF.

If you don't know what loving yourself means for you, just relax and keep reading—you'll understand and experience it more as this goes along. There's also a whole chapter on what loving yourself means in "In Your Self". Below you'll find a download for an extract which explains more about self-love.

"How can I love myself if my parents didn't love me?" you want to know.
"How can I love myself if I shout at my kids?"
"How can I love myself if I've perpetrated a crime?"
"How can I love myself if I don't have a partner/ if I'm a failure at business/ if my skin's this color/ if I let people down/ if I hurt others/ if my penis is too small/ if my breasts are droopy/ if I'm too fat/ if I'm not clever/ if I'm not normal/ if my best is not enough ...?"

I ask you, "How can you *not*?"

Let's talk about how to.

DOWNLOAD What does it mean to love yourself?
www.ifilovedmyself.com/members/chapter-1

DOWNLOAD Chapter 1 summary
www.ifilovedmyself.com/members/chapter-1

Chapter 2

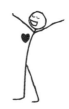

What the Love question reveals and why

"What I know for sure is that you feel real joy in direct proportion to how connected you are to living your truth."
Oprah Winfrey

"Find that truth, live that truth and everything else will come."
Ellen DeGeneres

Listen to your Truth—it knows stuff

Years ago I attended hypnotherapy training and the teacher mentioned that many people walk around with a sense of numbness—a kind of deadness inside that blocks real deep feeling and presence in life. We discussed various ways of using hypnotherapy to help people 'come alive' again. I remember standing outside during a tea break, gazing at a tree, thinking of my own areas of numbness that I'd simply accepted as normal for me, and thinking to myself in total amazement, *You can HEAL that?!*

Now, after years of exploring hypnotherapy, meditation, energy work and various forms of self-development, I hardly ever get that sense of numbness any more. I guess I got my answer: *Yes, you can heal that!* If numbness ever arises in me now, I'm very aware of it because it feels uncomfortable—not my usual feeling of being alive and present.

Much of what was underlying my own numbness—and that of so many people—was a disconnection between my heart and my Self and my Truth. Now if that numbness comes up, I understand it's showing me that I'm turning away from some Truth of mine; that somewhere I'm not letting myself listen to what my heart is feeling and needing. As soon as I notice it, I sit and have a chat with my heart and my Truth. (I'll explain how to do that in the next chapter.) The reassuring answers and wisdom I receive guide me in incredibly accurate ways.

Someone once asked me, "Why do you seem happy so much of the time?" and I replied, "I listen to myself." That's all each of us has to do to feel better and live the life we long for. I'm serious. If it sounds simple, that's because it is. If it sounds complicated or confusing, that's OK too—keep reading and it'll become clearer. I'm constantly amazed at how marvelous I feel my life is now and how it keeps getting better—simply because I practice self-love and listen to my feelings. I ask myself what I need and then take my needs seriously. If my needs are regularly quite well met, I'm bound to feel good, right? It's a simple formula. I've witnessed many of my clients master this and start to really enjoy their lives.

The part that's sometimes less simple is overcoming fears and resistance to making the life changes that our Truth requires and—believe it or not—fears and resistance to being happy. But fear not your fears! If you're willing to try this out but don't know how to, I'm thrilled to announce that you already have a built-in personal guidance system to take you through the process step by step in the best possible way for you. Any time you need help, you can access it by asking the Love question: *If I loved myself, what would I choose to do now?*

Asking this and listening for the answer is guaranteed to give you point-by-point guidance to where you most long to go. Chapter 3 explains exactly how to use this simple yet powerful question, but first, I'll give you some useful information to help you understand how and why it works.

The magic ingredient for loving yourself

Marshall Rosenberg, founder of the highly effective conflict-resolution method, Nonviolent Communication (NVC), emphasized the fact that we all have needs. When these needs are met, we feel good. When these needs are not met, we feel bad. It's a simple principle but we struggle with it—probably because we get distracted by feelings. We tend to focus on what we think is *causing* us to feel a certain way, rather than seeing that the feelings are merely *showing* us which of our needs are met or unmet in that moment.

Needs have gotten a bad rap in our individualistic society. We see them as weak, we don't like to admit we have them and it's not a compliment to call someone 'needy'. But we *do* all have them, and they are legitimate and even beautiful. Acknowledging our needs and values is an essential part of our own and our human community's health and well-being. NVC is probably so effective in easing conflict between parties precisely because it emphasizes respect for everyone's needs.

This book is not specifically associated with or promoting NVC—although it's definitely worth looking into if you want to learn how to communicate effectively and compassionately. I share this because the concept of needs is vital to listening to your Truth and loving yourself. It can be life-changing to turn your focus towards identifying your own needs. When you don't know what exactly is causing your upset or joy, you have no way of easing or prolonging it. Once you know what's happening at the core of your feelings, you can take loving and effective action.

Sometimes people feel confused about what a need actually is. I find it helpful to think of it like this:

When you need something, its absence makes you feel unsettled, distressed or dissatisfied to some degree. It feels

like something is wrong or missing in your world, as though things are not as they should be for you.

If your need is being met, you have a mild to intense sense of well-being. You feel pleased and content, like all is as it should be in your world.

I'll illustrate with an example. Let's say you've made a small effort for someone and you have a need for acknowledgement. If they don't acknowledge what you've done, you'll feel a little disgruntled, like something isn't there that should be. It feels uncomfortable, and is something you'll need to shake off to feel fully OK again. If, however, they do understand the effort you've made for them, you feel pleased and satisfied; as though things are right in your world. That's the mild version.

Now let's say you've made a great and sustained effort for someone or something, and you have a need for acknowledgement. Let's also say that not only are your efforts completely brushed aside, but others who did less than you are credited for *their* efforts and receive payment and promotion for *their* input. This will feel intensely uncomfortable for you. You'll feel a strong and urgent sense that something's wrong, something that should be there is missing. If, however, your need is met and your efforts are credited and acknowledged, you'll have a deep sense of satisfaction and well-being—a feeling that your life is on track and things are as they need to be.

Meeting your needs is the magic ingredient for satisfying self-loving.

Three simple ways to identify your needs

You understand if your dog whines restlessly because he needs a walk. You're not surprised if a plant wilts when its need for water isn't met. You don't expect a business to thrive if its needs for capital, initiative and dedicated people aren't met. You don't anticipate that people will be happy when a politician doesn't meet the needs of the constituency. All creatures and systems have needs for functioning well, yet somehow we expect *ourselves* to be fine even when our needs are not met.

You have to pay attention to your needs and make sure they are fulfilled if you want to thrive—it's a foundational rule for life.

One of the reasons the Love question works so well is that the answer often comes in the form of how you can meet your most pressing need of that moment.

Look at the list of needs on page 32 taken from the Center for Nonviolent Communication website (https://www.cnvc.org/Training/needs-inventory).

I remember feeling surprised the first time I read it by what are considered legitimate needs for every human. As you read through this list, think about how it might feel when that need is met and when it is not met.

LIST OF NEEDS

The following list is neither exhaustive nor definitive. It is meant as a starting place to support anyone who wishes to engage in a process of deepening self-discovery and to facilitate greater understanding and connection between people. (In this moment I/ they have a need for):

CONNECTION	PHYSICAL WELL-BEING	HONESTY	MEANING
acceptance	air	authenticity	awareness
affection	food	integrity	celebration of life
appreciation	movement/ exercise	presence	challenge
belonging	rest/sleep		clarity
cooperation	sexual expression	**PLAY**	competence
communication	safety	joy	consciousness
closeness	shelter	humour	contribution
community	touch		creativity
companionship	water		discovery
compassion		**PEACE**	efficacy
consideration	**AUTONOMY**	beauty	effectiveness
consistency	choice	communion	growth
empathy	freedom	ease	hope
inclusion	independence	equality	learning
intimacy	space	harmony	mourning
love	spontaneity	inspiration	participation
mutuality		order	purpose
nurturing			self-expression
respect/ self-respect			stimulation
safety			to matter
security			understanding
stability			
support			
to know and be known			
to see and be seen			
to understand and be understood			
trust			
warmth			

(c) 2005 by The Center for Nonviolent Communication
www.cnvc.org Email: cnvc@cnvc.org

How do you use this information? Any strong unpleasant feelings show you that a need of yours is not being met. Here are three simple ways to determine what your need is:

EXERCISE: IDENTIFYING YOUR NEED

- Ask yourself, "What do I need?" You can use the list opposite to help identify your need.
- Notice what you feel and ask yourself, "What's the opposite of that feeling?" If you feel disrespected, you have a need for respect. If you feel scared, you have a need for safety, etc.
- Ask the handy Love question.

Once you understand what you need, you can find a way to meet it. Being kind to yourself and identifying the needs beneath your strong feelings gives you the tools to communicate clearly and empathically with yourself and others.

But won't I be pampering myself?

Figuring out our *real* needs can be a little tricky at times. Sometimes we make choices that only *seem* loving but what we *think* we want or need is actually self-destructive. Sometimes we say, "Ah, who cares! If I loved myself, I'd watch a third episode of this series and eat ice cream, even though I know I'll feel tired and bloated tomorrow."

When we do self-destructive things, we *are* genuinely trying to meet our needs—maybe for fun and freedom, as in this case—but we're doing it in self-damaging ways. That's not actually self-love, even though it can look like it. The way to distinguish it is how it leaves you feeling. Good = it met the need. Bad = it didn't.

Self-destructive behavior is a call for help from ourselves to ourselves, and it only happens when our needs aren't being met in more direct and self-loving ways.

When we do self-destructive things, we're saying to ourselves, "My need to be nourished, affirmed and loved at the end of this challenging day is not being met. Maybe junk food/ wine/ TV/ cellphone/ porn/ cigarettes/ video games/ Internet/ my abusive partner will satisfy my need for love, care and nurturing and then I'll feel better."

Like children, we seek out something that will *seem* to meet our need. But when we see that the replacement is not the real thing, we come face to face with the painful absence of what we most want. A substitute for love, for example, usually leaves us feeling emptier than before.

We make hundreds or even thousands of decisions each and every day, and our real Self has an opinion about each of these. If our real needs are met, we feel good. If our real needs aren't met, we feel bad. How often do you stop to listen? Listening means feeling instantly better. So why don't we just listen all the time and feel good?

If you loved yourself, which of your needs would you attend to now?

This and the following exercise are possibly the two most important in this book

EXERCISE: ACTIVE SELF-LOVE

One of the most powerful ways you can love yourself is to actively say nice and loving things to yourself in your mind. Deliberately tell yourself the things you wish you heard from others. I recommend you start right now and never stop—ever. Once you try it and see how it feels, you'll understand why I say that. Here's how it might sound:

- "Good morning (name). It's lovely to be me this morning. I'm so glad I wake up to me every morning."
- "You're doing so well (name). I'm really pleased with you. Just because."
- "(Name), I really love you, you're wonderful."
- "Everything's OK as it is. I'm so pleased to be me."
- "I love how you try so hard (name), even though you're already just fine."
- "I am precious to me."
- "I like how I did that. Well done me!"
- "I love me, I love myself, I love you (name)"
- "I'm beautiful, no matter what."
- "I'm feeling a little rough today. That's OK. I can just feel how I feel and I'll love me and be kind to me and look after myself more because I'm feeling tender."
- "It's OK. I'm OK."

Say at least five kind things to yourself daily for a week and see what happens. I hope after that week, you never stop.

If you constantly say kind, loving and encouraging things to yourself inside your mind, you're going to feel loved and affirmed.

It makes life *a lot* easier and more pleasant and it's also extremely freeing. You'll be amazed how many needs are met that you usually seek to meet elsewhere.

How to feel your feelings

I often say, "Just stay with your feelings. Don't try to avoid your feelings—let yourself feel them." Sometimes people gaze at me blankly because they don't have any idea what this means or how to do it.

I wish there was a class in elementary school called 'How to be human'. This stuff needs to be learnt. So let's start:

Feelings are physical sensations. Anger, fear, boredom, etc, all begin with physical sensations (prickling heat, beating heart, numbness, dullness). What usually happens is that when we start to feel these sensations, a deep part of us understands that we're required to take an action. This is where we trip up.

The action your feeling is prompting you to take is to listen to your heart so that you live your Truth.

We misinterpret that prompt and look for what we're supposed to change about that moment—outside ourselves! Big mistake. It's *inside* ourselves we're supposed to be looking. But when we feel the physical sensations that indicate a message from our heart, we respond by trying to change our situation, our circumstances, or other peoples' behaviours or attitudes … That's when we end up blaming others, getting into arguments, being controlling, seeking to change our car/hair colour/body/clothes/partner because we think that's what will change the feelings we have. We totally miss the point. And our heart continues to let us know that something needs to change—but it's inside us, not outside.

Here's an exercise to help:

EXERCISE: HOW TO FEEL YOUR FEELINGS

Whenever you notice yourself having feelings—you're angry or anxious, distressed, stressed, bored, restless, uncertain—stop. Just stop whatever you're doing, wherever you are. Stop mid-sentence or mid-step and say, "Oh, I'm having feelings."

Then tune in to your body. Where do you feel any sensation? Where do you feel it most strongly?

- Do you feel movement—contracting, tightness, expanding, stirring—anywhere in your body?
- Do you feel temperature—heat, cold, neutral?
- Does it feel like a softening, opening, hardening, protecting …?
- Does it have a shape—spiky, square, spiral …?
- Do you sense a color that comes with the feeling?

All this is to help you become present to the feeling. Now, very importantly, stay with the sensations. Do not analyse what they might be or why they came. Just say, "Oh, this is how I feel. How interesting. Let me observe what's happening inside me."

As you remain open to the sensations, tears or sadness or emotional pain might bubble up. That's good! This is the real emotion beneath the physical sensations. Realisations may come with this. As best you can, stay still and allow these emotions to come up and out. This is the real You. It's your Truth.

Do your best to stay in the moment, in the feelings, observing instead of trying to explain or justify the feelings.

However you are able to, say kind, accepting and loving things to yourself while this is happening, as if you're a child you loved. Stay in it as long as it lasts. Don't worry, it doesn't last long. Try it and see.

Feelings that are fully allowed to be felt tend to flower and fade quite quickly and leave a sense of clarity and peace.

Feelings that are avoided can last a lifetime and cause a lot of havoc.

If you loved yourself, what feeling would you let yourself feel now?

How to feel better immediately

People often say, "You don't get a rule book for life." This isn't strictly true. We actually come fully equipped with an amazing guidance system, but we tend to ignore it as we stumble around, feeling miserable and complaining about how hard and pointless life is. When we *do* listen, life becomes smoother and easier, and we feel better—even in hard times—because our needs are being met.

Our guidance system comes with a built-in alarm that alerts us to when we aren't listening to ourselves. (For more on this, see Chapter 5, "If I loved myself in my body and health", and the chapter on thoughts and feelings in "In Your Self"). This alarm uses our feelings to let us know whether we are on or off track, and it's highly effective: when you feel bad in any way, you're off track, and when you feel good in any way, you're on track. Could it be any simpler than that? A child could follow it. In fact, children do—and they follow their feelings a lot better than grown-ups do, because somewhere along the line we adults were told not to listen to our own guidance system and rely on the outside for direction. In the immortal words of Julia Roberts's character in the film *Pretty Woman* to the sales lady who didn't serve her: "Big mistake. Big. HUGE!" When we don't recognize the beauty, quality and wealth of our Truth and when we refuse to give it service, we lose out—big time.

When we listen to ourselves in real ways, we start to feel loved. We feel important enough to be listened to, which implies we are worthy and good enough, and that's what we're all seeking. It's very simple:

When you listen to yourself and follow what you need, you feel good. When you listen to outside opinions for your life decisions or ignore your inner guidance, you feel bad.

That's it. I could end this book right here. Everything I say from here onwards is just a variation on or example of this simple idea. But to put it into practice in a daily, real-life way takes repetition. Most of us are so well trained in not listening to ourselves that a whole book is necessary to help us come back to our true nature. I *wrote* this book and I still have to remind myself to do this! You and I are worthy, lovable, important, good-enough beings who know exactly what feels right and good for us.

It's not always so easy though, is it? Especially when we're feeling fear of some kind. The next section explains why.

If you loved yourself, what would you choose to do now?

Some neuroscience behind decision-making: from fear or love

When we perceive something in our environment as threatening, our bodies are designed to deal with it in the good old caveman way: kill it, run away from it or stand completely still hoping it won't see us. That's the fight-flight-freeze response that stress experts always talk about.

A comprehensive physiological process occurs to help the body do what it needs to do to survive. Adrenalin surges through the body giving muscles extra strength and stamina, the heart pumps faster bringing more blood to the lungs and muscles—an entire chemical and mechanical extravaganza goes on in our complex and brilliant systems to facilitate our staying alive and unharmed. Part of the flurry of activity in response to (real or perceived) danger is that our cognitive functioning shifts. Our higher analytic processes briefly shut down in order to help us act decisively in a moment of threat. There's a parable about this:

> **THE FOX AND THE CAT**
>
> An arrogant fox asked a cat, "What would you do if a hunter was to come along now?"
> "I'd run straight up a tall tree and hide," the cat answered.
> The fox laughed derisively. "Is that all you've got? Well, I might do that, but I could also run beneath that bush, or hide behind a thick tree trunk, or dash to that field over there, or into my burrow over yonder. I have many more options than you!"
> At that very moment a hunter arrived. Within seconds the cat had bolted up a tall tree to hide amongst the leaves. The fox stood deliberating which of his many clever escape plans to choose—and the hunter went home with a handsome new fox fur.

If you see a truck barreling towards you at high speed, what would you instinctively do? Jump out of its way as fast as possible, right? People who've had experiences like this will often say afterwards, "I don't even remember how I got out of the way. It happened so fast."

In a time of real immediate threat or crisis, our brain shuts down analytic processing and shifts to our reptilian-brain response.

Evolution seems to have helped us lose the trait of contemplating in these situations. Quick as a lizard we take action—often with life-saving results. Then, as our brain comes back online, we begin to analyze what happened.

Interestingly, one of the life-saving reactions to threat is disorganized behavior. An animal under threat will sometimes begin running chaotically this way and that. They literally 'run around in a blind panic'. Sometimes disorganized behavior can get the animal into trouble (precisely because it's unthinking) but many more times it saves them: it's much more difficult for a predator to catch prey moving quickly in an unpredictable pattern.

When we're in an emotional space of fear, our physiological system responds in the same way it does to a physical threat. Your body can't distinguish between the fear you feel in response to facing a lion or to facing your partner leaving you. A threat is a threat, and your body will start the process to help you survive: to fight, flee, freeze or run around in chaos. And while those things can help with our physical survival, you just need to think of how a person may react to their loved one leaving them to note that these reactions aren't always constructive for our social survival—and our humiliation. Sure we stay alive—success, according to our brain—but we may wish we hadn't.

It makes sense that when we're faced with a decision of any kind—be it changing jobs, having a child or reacting to a colleague's comment—we would want to make sure that we have all of our cognitive faculties online. This isn't the case if we're experiencing fear of any kind, which is one of the big reasons that decisions we make from places of fear often turn out unhappily.

"OK, so I won't make big decisions while I'm freaking out," you may say. The thing is, much of the time we don't even realize we are being motivated by fear rather than, for example, love and trust. And we may not even realize we're freaking out.

Most of the time we're nudged along by two kinds of motivation: fear and desire.

We tend to be either chased from behind or drawn forward to something. An example of fear: "If I don't speak nicely to my whining, irritating, totally irrational child/colleague, I will be a bad parent/person." An example of desire: "I want to be connected to the love that is me so I choose to speak kindly to my whining, irritating, totally irrational child/colleague."

The behavior may look exactly the same from the outside, but the internal experiences are vastly different. When a choice is fear-driven, you feel accomplishment or relief when you complete the task, but you're also on the lookout for the next threat. Being motivated by desire is like walking towards yourself: you feel open, at ease and pleased with yourself. In the first case, your body is bombarded with stress chemicals and hormones like cortisol and adrenaline, which feel unpleasant and shut down your brain. In the second, you are flooded with love chemicals like oxytocin, norepinephrine and dopamine, which make you feel relaxed, connected and joyful.

Our decisions are affected by our state of mind—we are more open to new things when happy than when we are depressed or afraid.

Therefore, the kinds of decisions you make in one state or the other can have vastly different outcomes.

When you regularly check in with your heart, you trigger the regular release of love chemicals. Besides being extremely beneficial to your health, these help you live in a way that is more desire-driven and this will better benefit you in the grand scheme of your life. So this loving yourself thing is important to learn how to do if you want to make satisfying decisions.

EXERCISE: HOW TO MAKE A DECISION IN THE MIDST OF FEAR

If you need to make a decision in the midst of fear, try first to pause and connect with your heart. It can help in these times to think of your heart as a small child or a cute, fluffy baby animal in the center of your chest. Take a number of slow deep breaths, letting the air go right into your lower abdomen.
Then ask:
- If I loved myself, what would I choose to do now?
- If I knew I was safe, what would I choose to do now?
- If I had no fear, what would I choose to do now?

Is this for everyone?

I hope at this point you feel motivated to try the Love question. If however you feel you just *can't* love yourself, please keep reading.

No one is excluded from the idea of loving themselves and following their own Truth—no matter what.

Our human world is wonderful in many ways, but it's not fair and it's not always kind or easy. Some people have a much harder journey to loving themselves than others. If things have happened in your life that make you dislike yourself, for example, or your community deems you 'different' in some way. Or you feel shamed just for being who you are—this can make loving yourself more challenging. Being targeted for abuse, or the different one in your family, poor amongst the rich, dark-skinned in a light-skin-dominant culture, disabled in an abled setting, female in a male-dominated space, having a learning difficulty amongst highly literate people, or being homosexual in a homophobic environment can make you feel like you have no real right to exist. I share powerful stories about people facing some of these issues in "In Your Self". There are myriad ways we can be treated, by ourselves and others, that do not meet our needs or affirm our worth or our lovability. It can be very hard to love yourself when the pervasive message is: *Who you are is not acceptable. You don't fit in; you're not good enough; you don't have as much worth as others.*

"The most potent weapon in the hands of the oppressor is the mind of the oppressed."

Steve Biko's immortal words in *"I Write What I Like"*, 1978, tap into the core of this issue. If you believe you're not as good as others, you'll keep yourself oppressed. No one will need to tell you to stay in line: you'll shame *yourself* into not shining your true Self. But that's not self-loving—or true.

It's more difficult to respect and meet your deeper needs when you're not shown respect in your surroundings. Even if you *know* it's not true, part of you might still wonder if you're somehow 'less' and that makes it harder to love and listen to yourself. Even though feeling uncomfortable or ashamed of things about yourself over which you have no control can weaken your self-confidence, it doesn't mean you don't get to honor your Truth. We all have the right to have our needs met.

When a successful person from a marginalised group is interviewed, they often talk about the difficult circumstances they faced. Their message is frequently a version of: *You are not your circumstances. Don't let your past dictate who you are now. Don't give other people the power to decide for you.* They've found ways of not allowing their minds to be oppressed. They've managed to love themselves enough to listen to their Truth.

If you experience circumstances in which you are subject to prejudice, aggression or disregard, self-love might feel like something for those who 'fit in'. But it's for *everyone*—whether society says we're 'ideal' or not.

Only you know what your real deeper needs and values are. Make it your quest to ensure your needs are met so you can thrive and shine your true Self. We'll all be better for it.

If you ever feel downhearted or unworthy and unloved, let your love come from the source that is You. You have every right to do so—the world needs you to love yourself—and you'll feel happier and more empowered. Walk your own path of love and worth in those tough moments by asking:

If I loved myself, what would I choose to do now?

 Pause now, take a breath and say something kind to yourself

What will this Love question give me?

The answers you receive from the Love question offer a compassionate response to yourself in times of joy as well as times of need and distress.

Asking yourself the Love question, even in truly desperate moments and circumstances, is the beginning of finding your way towards whatever is best for you.

No one but you can say what that 'best' might be. In fact, *you* might not even know that yet. The answers to the Love question are often surprising—I explain this more in Chapter 3. You might choose to stay in situations you thought you wanted to escape—but with a completely different perspective. Or things you thought were serving you may show themselves to be acts of self-sabotage.

Your heart's answer is never something unrealistic or unmanageable for you. It'll also never be something that keeps you 'small' or limited to what's comfortable for society. Your Truth will gently guide you to where your heart longs to be—which is also where you'll best be of benefit to the world.

Using the Love question probably won't provide immediate solutions to large-scale institutional problems (besides the most obvious and important one that if we each loved ourselves, prejudice and power games would no longer exist). You cannot expect the Love question to instantly 'fix' a disempowering situation (although occasionally it might).

WHAT THE LOVE QUESTION REVEALS AND WHY

> **ASKING YOURSELF THE LOVE QUESTION WILL:**
>
> - introduce and affirm the notion that loving yourself is an action;
> - suggest that you have permission to ask your own opinion;
> - offer the idea that your opinion is the most useful one for you to listen to for all of your life choices;
> - help you see what your needs are and how best to meet them;
> - give you real, manageable steps and guidance to begin changing both how you feel about any situation and what to do about it;
> - help you listen to and trust your own Truth;
> - enhance your experience of feeling safe and loved in the world;
> - suggest that you have reasons and the right to love yourself;
> - begin an internal conversation about what works for you and what doesn't;
> - bring awareness to the discomfort you might feel in a situation and clarity as to its causes;
> - make you realize at some point that your lovability and worth are inherent and have nothing to do with anything that has happened to you from outside;
> - shift your power away from the external situation or people, and place it firmly in your own hands.

Are you ready to learn how to use this magical Love question? Then turn the page and let's do this!

Welcome to your Truth-led life.

DOWNLOAD Chapter 2 summary
www.ifilovedmyself.com/members/chapter-2

A NOTE ON THE WORD 'LOVE'

For many of us the word 'love' is loaded with meanings—some good, some bad. You might have a visceral reaction to the word, which can get in the way of using the Love question comfortably. If you find yourself asking, "But what is love anyway?" or, "I have an issue with love," or, "I don't know how to love properly," know that these challenges are dealt with throughout the book.

You can, however, choose to use another word that suits you better. If you decide to use an alternative word to 'love' in your question, I suggest that every once in a while you return to the original wording—to 'love'—to see if and how your feelings have changed.

Here are some alternatives to using the word 'love'—feel free to add your own:

- If I was in alignment with my true Self, what would I choose to do now?
- If I knew I had permission to take up space, what would I choose to do now?
- How would I best meet my needs now?
- If I knew I was OK as I am, what would I choose to do now?
- If I had no fear, what would I choose to do now?
- If I knew everyone else would be OK, what would I choose to do now?
- If I knew everyone else also loved themselves, what would I choose to do now?
- If I knew it was OK to shine, what would I choose to do now?
- If I knew everyone had enough, what would I choose to do now?
- If I liked myself, what would I choose to do now?
- If I knew I was safe, what would I choose to do now?

Using these versions in addition to the Love question can be enriching, so you can view these as complimentary guiding questions to finding your best path in any moment.

Chapter 3

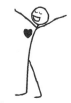

How to use the Love question

"Follow your heart, and listen when it speaks to you."
Susanna Tamaro

The most effective way to ask the Love question

In our psychotherapy session one day, Ezra is asking the Love question and becoming very frustrated. The answers he's receiving are what he usually hears in his head. His head knows what he 'should' do to be more healthy, and when he asks himself the Love question he's getting answers like, "If I loved myself, I'd exercise more," or, "I'd eat better." While these answers are true in a practical sense, I can see he's feeling downhearted, shamed and discouraged because those are things he already knows—and is already failing at. He looks tired and despondent. This is not how your personal Truth makes you feel.

Your Truth may surprise you, but when you hear it, you *know* it deep within yourself. Your chest softens and opens up, and you feel inspired by relief and hope.

Ezra is not looking inspired in any way.

To help him ease into it I explain, "This technique is not about asking the questions to which your head already knows the answers. Those answers come with the flavor of 'I should ...' They're generally not happy-feeling answers. This question is about asking your heart what it wants. Expect the unexpected."
"I think I confuse my head with me," he replies.

So we try the Love question again. This time, I ask him to become conscious of being himself by adding a precursor: "I am Ezra, sitting here now, facing this choice."
Then he really feels into his heart space (more on that shortly) and asks, "If I loved myself, if I was someone who loves himself, what would I choose to do now?"

The answer comes quite suddenly: "I wouldn't be so hard on myself. I'd go slow." And then a beatific smile spreads across his face as he relaxes into the chair.
"Oh," he says after a few moments of peaceful silence, "is that how this works?"

Yes, that's how this works.

An answer from your heart is immediately soothing and reassuring.

The other day I woke up full of plans and thoughts and feeling pressure to get them done. It didn't feel good. So I sat down to meditate and ask myself the Love question that I knew would guide me to my best next step. At first I got a head answer: *If I loved myself, I'd get these things done because then I'll feel better.*

But I didn't feel any relief. I still felt tension. So I checked in with myself: "I am Eilat, sitting here right now, feeling this stress. If I loved myself, what would I choose to do now?"

The answer came very quickly: "I'd be gentle with myself." It came with a knowing that everything was OK and that I was doing fine. My chest softened and opened. All of a sudden, I felt relaxed and reassured; everything was better. It's the same feeling we get when we're having a difficult moment and someone we trust tells us everything's going to be fine.

When you ask yourself the Love question, you get that feeling from the part of you—your heart—that will take every opportunity to tell you that you're OK.

When we take the time to listen to our heart, we get constant loving reassurance, which makes life a whole lot easier to deal with.

How to ask from a heart space

"I am [say your name]. I am here in this situation right now. If I loved myself, what would I choose to do now?"

The Love question will not work when you're in a space of judgment, because judgment comes from your head.

Your head only knows how to make the decision that looks the *safest*—not the *best*—for you. The answer you seek comes from the heart.

This is as true for lighter decisions, like what to eat for breakfast, as for serious situations, like how to extract yourself from an abusive relationship. Even if you're angry at someone or something for putting you in a position where you have to make the decision, judging and blaming yourself or someone else is *not* going to help you make the choice that *feels* best to you.

When you're facing a decision on how to move forward, be still for a moment and let the situation be what it is. We often check out of ourselves when we feel threatened. Instead, take a slow deep breath and try to become present in your body. Be aware that you are inside your body, looking out from your own eyes. Notice how your body feels, any areas of tension or tightness. Notice where and how you're standing or sitting. Become aware of your feet on the ground. Then, without analysing it too much, simply acknowledge the choice facing you.

Be in acceptance for a moment: *This is what it is.*

Now ask the question: *If I loved myself, what would I choose to do now?*

We may struggle to make decisions because we have expectations of ourselves and our lives. Whenever you ask the Love question, don't assume you already know the answer. Expect the unexpected. I've often burst out in surprised laughter—or tears—when I've received my answer. We might avoid making decisions:

- for fear of losing someone or something,
- for fear of looking foolish,
- because we're wanting to please others, or
- because we're clinging to a certain way of seeing ourselves.

The beautiful part of the Love question is that your heart knows exactly who you are, what you fear and what will help you feel better. And the answer is often unexpected.

For example, trying to decide whether to leave your job is a huge, life-changing decision. You may be afraid your heart will say you should leave because you *know* you've been unhappy there for a long time. But that's your head talking. On asking the Love question, the heart response is, "Start playing music again."

What? That doesn't feel like an answer—except that when you hear it, your chest softens and opens as you remember how much you love playing music, and you suddenly feel relieved and hopeful about good times ahead.

Even though work sucks, I can at least enjoy my music, you reassure yourself. And later it may unfold that you meet some new people through your music. As you move into a better space doing more things you love, you're less troubled by the challenges at work. You feel less desperate, so you're open when you meet someone who needs your exact skills. And it all works out organically that you leave your job and you even feel a bit sad saying goodbye because your life has improved.

But that's all later. At the beginning, all you hear is, "Start playing music again."

Trust what you hear if you *feel* relief from the answer you get.

You'll know it's your Truth because it'll make deep sense to you, even if you can't put it into words. Hearing your Truth makes things feel lighter and better, and it comes with a deep, relaxing breath and a feeling of, *Oh, everything is actually OK.*

> **EXERCISE:** **LISTENING TO YOUR HEART TRUTH**

To review the process:
1. Become aware of yourself in your body and say your name: "I am …"
2. Acknowledge the facts of the situation you are in, without judging it.
3. Ask the question, *If I loved myself, what would I choose to do now?*
4. Listen and pay attention to how the answer *feels*. If it brings a sense of opening, relief and joy, you know it's your heart's answer, your Truth. If not, see what happens when you ask again. And again.

Be gentle and kind to yourself as you try—whether or not it works straight away.

This is easier to do with small decisions at first, but by practising listening to your heart, even complex and emotion-filled decisions will become easier to make in a way that leaves you feeling at peace with yourself.

Practise feeling a heart answer

I want to teach you how to listen for your heart Truth. You'll need five to ten minutes in which you won't be interrupted. (If you can't do this now, mark the page and do it later when you have time to try it out.)

> **EXERCISE:** **HOW DOES A HEART ANSWER FEEL?**

Turn your attention inwards. Allow your body to relax. Take a slow deep breath in, hold it for a moment and then slowly release it. Become aware of your breathing. Don't try to change it in any way; simply observe your breath

HOW TO USE THE LOVE QUESTION

entering and leaving your body. Do this for about three breath cycles—in and out—and then read on.

Now think of the word 'yes'. Let 'yes' float around inside you, and notice what you begin to feel. How does your chest feel when you think 'yes'? How does your body feel? What kind of energy is flowing inside you when you feel the word 'yes'? Notice areas in your body that are particularly tense or relaxed in response to the word. Stay with this for a minute or two (or longer if you're enjoying it). When you're ready, read on.

Let that go, and simply notice your breath again for three cycles of in and out breaths.

Next, bring the word 'no' to your mind. As with 'yes', let 'no' float around inside you and notice what you begin to feel. How does your chest feel when you think 'no'? How does your body feel? What kind of energy is flowing inside you when you feel the word 'no'? Notice areas in your body that are particularly tense or relaxed in response to the word. Read on when that feels complete.

Let that go, and simply notice your breath again for three cycles of in and out breaths.

Bring the word 'maybe' to your mind. Let 'maybe' float around inside you and notice what you begin to feel. How does your chest feel when you think 'maybe'? How does your body feel? What kind of energy is flowing inside you when you feel the word 'maybe'? Notice areas in your body that are particularly tense or relaxed in response to the word.

Let that go, and simply notice your breath again for three cycles of in and out breaths.

Ponder what you've just experienced. You probably noticed that each word brings its own physical and mental experience.

Remember now how 'yes' feels. Your heart Truth feels like the word 'yes'— and then some. Sometimes you'll feel it strongly and sometimes subtly, but 'yes' is the feeling you're looking for when listening for your heart response.

If it's one of the other feelings, that's not it yet. Keep asking.

If you didn't feel much in this exercise, don't worry. Your heart knows how to contact you in a way that will make sense to you. All you need to do is be open to it and listen.

The job descriptions of your head and your heart

I would like to properly introduce you now to Head and Heart—two characters that are vital to understanding how this 'If I loved myself' question works. Head and Heart are an odd pairing—they have such different ways about them—but when they partner up there are none that can beat them.

Heart is a wonderful character who's all about feelings and desire and inspiration. Heart is happiest when it can play and be open to the world and other people. It's always on the lookout for where it will be happiest. Heart has excellent internal hearing and is constantly scanning the space you're in, listening for the melody that it finds most beautiful. Heart has a keen ability to hear the melody that resonates most clearly with its highest Truth. As soon as it recognizes the purest notes, it's drawn to wherever the melody is coming from: "There, there—I want to go there! That's where the melody is. That's what feels best to me." Heart wants nothing more than to move towards what feels good.

The problem is that while it has phenomenal capacity for inner hearing, Heart doesn't have very good external vision. While it can hear the beautiful melody and knows where it wants to go, it can't really see how to get there, and it can't get there on its own. Left to its own devices, Heart will bumble and blunder, make illogical decisions and embark on confusing paths. You know when they say 'Love is blind' …

HOW TO USE THE LOVE QUESTION

This is where Head comes in.

Oh, Head! What a marvelous, upstanding character. Such excellent external vision, so clear and logical. In any given situation, Head can easily see the best way to go. One might think that all decisions should be left up to Head, but if Head is left to its own devices, it will usually go the straightforward route. It will choose what seems most reasonable, rational and safe. "What's the problem?" you might ask. "It sounds wonderful. Much less messy."

The problem is that Head lacks Heart's powerful internal hearing: Head can't hear the beautiful melody that gets Heart so excited. This might not seem like a big deal—after all, rational decisions are usually good ones, right? Perhaps, but anyone who has a chosen a career that'll make money over the one that fulfills their passion will tell you that following Head alone comes at the cost of happiness, fulfillment, a sense of purpose, inspired creativity and contentment. That's a high price. Letting Head make the decisions on its own usually leads to an unhappy Heart and interestingly, it also doesn't make Head happy.

If Head has to make decisions without Heart's guidance, it becomes stressed. While it does love being in charge of a mission, Head doesn't thrive without first being given a target by Heart. Imagine leading a mission but not knowing where you're supposed to go—that's a recipe for fear and doubt. Like anyone with too much or inappropriate responsibility, Head begins to shut down, becoming anxious and rigid.

Like any couple, if Head and Heart disregard each other's needs and skills, they become unhappy and unbalanced. But when they work together, they're magnificent! Heart scans for and finds the melody: "There it is! There!" it calls out in excitement.

Head looks to see where Heart is pointing and (after sometimes sighing in exasperation) takes charge: "OK, let's see how we can get there. We have to move around that obstacle, build a raft to cross the river and follow that path. Off we go." Head puts its guiding hands on Heart's shoulders and they begin to move together towards the melody.

Every once in a while, Head asks Heart, "Now where?"

Heart listens for the melody, finds it, smiles happily and points. "That way!"

Head looks around for the most logical way to get there and off they go again.

Heart doesn't care how long it takes or what the route is—it's just so happy to be following the melody. Heart doesn't really care about outcomes or productivity—it cares only that whatever it's doing is in tune with its highest Truth and well-being. Heart is already living in its melody, already happy and content and full of purpose on the journey.

Head is equally relaxed and content fulfilling its role of helping Heart on its journey. It's stressful for Head to make decisions on its own because it knows vital information is missing. If a decision takes the pair away from Heart's melody, Head is affected by Heart's distress.

When we feel confused or distressed about a decision, this is the dynamic: Head or Heart are trying to make a decision without the other one, who keeps butting in.

When the two work in harmony, regardless of productivity or outcome, they feel fulfilled, excited and full of joy and purpose. 'Success' is an irrelevant concept in this scenario. The irony is that when you do what makes you happy, you tend to do it well and success follows ... but, critically, happiness comes first.

Listening with your heart and then allowing your head to show the way is the key to both happiness and success in all areas of your life.

This book is about learning to live life this way. Listening with your heart and following with your head and being happy, *happy*, HAPPY while you go along. Oh, and of course being successful and productive and having good relationships and everything else—but those are just the side-effects of happiness.

Here's a recipe for a happy life: Do everything in the way that makes your heart happy. Do nothing that makes your heart unhappy. And if you *have* to do something you're not excited to do, ask your heart how to do it in a way that will feel happiest and do it that way.

So how do you feel? Does the idea of doing this in your life make you a little nervous or excited? Nervousness is also normal. I'll explain.

Sometimes listening to your heart feels scary

There are times—especially at the start of this journey—when your heart tells you where it wants to go and it is *so* not what you'd planned for your life. It goes against logic, it suggests letting go of goals you've sweated over for years, it threatens your life as you know it.

If you've lived your life listening to your head, then chaos may ensue when you begin listening to your heart. If that makes you want to stop right here, I totally understand. This is a challenging concept and most of us don't really want to turn our life upside down. Maybe you're thinking: I have a good job. I have security and income. My spouse is nice enough (and who can expect romance after being married for this long?). I'm happy enough. The kids bring me some joy. I have some friends; we do nice things. Of course I have the feeling that there should be more to life than this, but everyone feels like that, don't they? We all have dreams when we're children—then we grow up. That's just life. I shouldn't want more. I mean, what am I going to do? Quit my job and become an artist like I always dreamed? Who would pay the bills? What would people say?

I get it. I really do. Most of us have compromised on our dreams in some way or another. And it's usually OK; it's something we can live with. But pause for a second ...
How's your heart doing?

Do you know, or are you afraid to ask it? As Dr Phil the TV shrink likes to ask, "How's that workin' for ya?"

One day I ask Dana, who's pregnant and in an unhappy relationship, to ask herself the Love question. She struggles to get an answer that gives her a 'yes' feeling. She stays in her head and gives rational responses that don't bring her any sense of Truth and no relief.
After a few tries, I ask her, "What are you blocking?"
She bursts into tears. "What if I hear I must leave the relationship?"

Her reaction makes complete sense. The consequences of ending a relationship are significant, and are even scarier when you're pregnant. If we've been making rational choices that override our heart's desires, then we tend to be afraid of what we may hear when we actually listen to ourselves.

The funny thing is that in many cases we already know when we're not being truthful with ourselves.

HOW TO USE THE LOVE QUESTION

"Is that what your heart is saying?" I ask Dana.
"I'm almost sure of it," she replies.

We don't continue with the exercise, but we'll get to it one day soon. Dana feels certain of what she'll hear but I'm not so sure, because when it comes to answers from the heart, I've learned to expect the unexpected.

Here's a personal example of hearing an unexpected heart Truth. The other day I had a long list of things to do and was feeling that my time was limited. Then my partner asked if I could run an errand for him. My initial head response was, *No, I can't. I have so much to do and if I say yes, I won't get to everything I'd like to finish.* Instead I took a deep breath and told him that I'd let him know later in the day.

Later, when it was time to do his errand, my head was still telling me that I should say no. His errand wasn't vital, and I had a lot to get through. It was a no-brainer, but I felt conflicted. So I stopped to check in and asked, "If I loved myself, what would I choose to do now?"

The immediate answer that came to me, along with my chest opening and my body relaxing, was, "Help him because I love him." I was so surprised—it wasn't at all what I'd expected, because I'd thought self-care would take the form of me doing my own thing. In that moment, however, self-care was not about keeping myself separate, but rather supporting my loved one and therefore increasing our intimacy. I did the errand and felt very pleased with myself for contributing to this relationship that is so precious to me. I felt loved by me for doing his errand in the middle of my busy day. How weird is that?!

Expect the unexpected. When I next ask Dana to listen to her heart Truth, even though she's afraid her heart will tell her to leave, the message may be something completely different. What I know for sure is that it will be a wise and kind answer.

While our head can be clever, it's not always wise. Real, deep wisdom requires the heart's input, because the heart knows our real needs. Clever choices are unsatisfying if the heart has had no say in the decision—and it's never wise to make a decision without all the information.

To gather that vital information from yourself, ask the Love question. Make sure when you do so that you're listening for a heart response, not a head one. If it's your heart responding, you'll *feel* it. You'll *feel* 'yes'. You'll *feel* love and reassurance and hope. You can't fake that feeling. It's either there or it isn't. Your needs are either met or they're not.

When you get a heart response, somehow everything inside you falls into place. So if Dana does ever get the message to leave the relationship, it'll come in a way that makes her feel safe and inspired.

 Pause now, take a breath and say something kind to yourself

Start small

You don't have to make huge life changes to begin listening with your heart.

You can begin simply with your everyday choices. In fact, the only place to begin making your life immediately more joyful is right this very moment.

These daily dilemmas may even seem silly:

- What shall I drink while I'm reading my book—the wine that relaxes me, but makes me feel heavy and a bit numb, or a cup of tea, which I find

soothing and which leaves me feeling lighter?
- Which route should I take to work—the longer beach road that lifts my spirits, or the quicker one through the city that leaves me feeling grey but saves time?
- What should I eat for lunch—the comforting food that leaves me feeling bloated, or the healthier, energising option?
- Should I pay attention to my partner/child or turn to this book I've been longing to read?

It may look as though there's a right and wrong choice to each question, but there isn't. It depends on your needs at that time. Some days one choice will feel good to you, and on another day it will be another that brings you a resounding 'yes'—even if you chose the junk food! (Chapter 6, "If I loved myself in my Food", explains why sometimes the less healthy option might be a Truth choice.)

The 'right' answer for you depends on the exact constellation of factors in that very moment. If you've already paid a lot of attention to your child and are now really needing quiet time, turning to your book will feel right and will benefit everyone. If you're avoiding intimacy and connection with your child, turning to your book will feel wrong and you can expect some hurt feelings and flaring tempers. Same answer, different outcomes. That's why this is a moment-by-moment adventure.

You'll find that as you listen with your heart in your daily decision-making is that you begin to feel more loved and cared for. This tends to have wonderful consequences for everyone, because your heart's sole task is to listen for *your* melody, the one that feels sweetest; that's the one where your needs are met. Your heart will never suggest something that's against your highest good. It also won't suggest anything that's unachievable.

When you do start to listen to your heart, the things you 'hear' might make you exclaim, "What?! I can't do *that*!" But if it's your heart saying it, you can and your happiness lies that way. You may not be able to fathom how to get there at first, but that will take care of itself.

It's a process to learn to listen with your heart and follow with your head.

Take one small step and one tiny decision at a time.

You'll find yourself crossing great distances and obstacles with surprising ease. And each time you turn towards your heart's melody, your heart will be happy, happy, happy.

Imagine walking around every day with a happy heart? Now that's worth it. Are you ready to learn how to apply the Love question everywhere?

Part Two will show you how.

DOWNLOAD Chapter 3 summary
www.ifilovedmyself.com/members/chapter-3

PART TWO

YOU CAN MASTER SELF-LOVE EVERYWHERE IN YOUR LIFE

What now?

Now we'll put this simple idea of the Love question to good use. The chapters in Part Two offer you more stories from my therapy room and my own life, along with some theory and neuroscience to support you in loving yourself in every area of your life (in particular work, money, your body, food, sex and parenting). In "In Your Self", relationships, thoughts and feelings, saying no, being and saying yes to life are covered.

Use the code or link at the start of each chapter to do the video meditation which helps you set an intention for the chapter to benefit you even more powerfully. The downloads of some of the exercises and chapter summaries are for you to print out and put in places you feel will support you (fridge, wall, etc.) At the end of the chapter, you may want to do the video meditation again to set your intention for going forward in that area of your life.

If you'd like to work with me in person or join one of my workshops or groups, follow this link or go to my website to find out how.

www.ifilovedmyself.com/work-with-eilat

From here on you can read the chapters in any order you wish. You might follow the book's layout and read in sequence, or you may want to turn back to the Contents page and find the chapter that feels most relevant to you. I suggest that you make sure to eventually read all the chapters, even if you don't feel they're directly relevant to your experience. Read the parenting section even if you're not a parent, for example—sometimes the tools and insights we need await us in the most surprising places.

If you're unsure of what to do at any point, just ask yourself the Love question and follow your heart.

Chapter 4

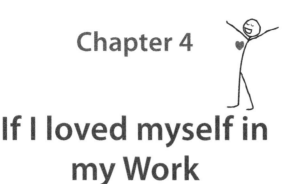

If I loved myself in my Work

Follow your bliss.
Joseph Campbell

SET AN INTENTION FOR THIS CHAPTER NOW

Setting an intention is a powerful way of increasing the effectiveness of what you are doing. Your intention is about your own needs and desired outcomes; it's unique to you and where you are in your life right now. Examples might be:
- My intention while reading this chapter is to see my patterns and choices that don't serve me at work and how to do things differently
- I have the intention to love and value myself at work
- I intend to learn how to meet my needs more while at work.

Before you work through the chapter, scan this code to join me for a short video meditation about setting an intention for yourself and your work.

You can also access the meditation through this link:
www.ifilovedmyself.com/members/chapter-4

Can you love yourself at work?

Can you imagine loving yourself at work? I hope you already do. At work—like anywhere else—what will serve you best is whatever flows from your answers to the Love question and variations like, *What do I need right now? How can I best love myself in this moment?*

We spend such a large part of our time at work, and yet we often compartmentalise it: there is Work and there is Me. It's hard enough to listen to ourselves *at all*, never mind at work. We say, "I can do this listening-to-myself-and-my-Truth, self-love stuff in my personal life, but at work I need to just get on with it. I have things to do. It's not about me and my needs."

As children we were largely taught that other people knew what was best for us. That was seldom true when we were children—you might remember feeling frustrated that your parents didn't understand what you really needed—and it's even less true when we're adults.

A child who's told, "Follow your dream, do what you love, find your passion..." is more likely to grow up to be successful and happy because she's been taught to make choices that feel good to her and to follow what feels right—for her. Unsurprisingly, such children's paths tend to be more joy-filled. Most of us were not taught that though, which is why we need to learn it later in life.

This whole book is about undoing the fallacy that someone else knows better than you what's best for you. Generally, if someone suggests they know you better than you do it's because they want you to stay in line—*their* line. Usually you can sense if the message is coming to you with care or with coercion. The first inspires respect, the second resentment.

At work, most of us are wary of crossing lines because, at the most basic level, we risk losing our source of income.

Being unhappy at your workplace does not serve you, your colleagues or your employers—it's in everyone's best interest that you find out and pursue what *does* make you happy.

This *may* mean leaving your job, but more often it means learning to do things differently *at* your current job. Self-love often comes down to small choices that make big differences to you moment by moment.

Always start with the small changes and choices—what unfolds from making truthful little changes can sometimes resolve the big problems in surprising ways.

If you stay aware of what feels right to you and make sure your needs are consistently met, you'll feel fulfilled *at work*. Imagine that.

Obvious ways to love yourself at work

This might seem odd, but I find it needs to be said:

You don't stop being a person while you're at work. You remain a person with needs and preferences wherever you go.

Bosses and employees alike tend to put their needs aside on 'work time'—and when they do, they can become ill and unhappy.

Labor law activists fought hard to secure the rights of workers to have tea and lunch breaks and reasonable working hours. They did this to prevent abuse of workers' time and energy. So ask yourself:

IF YOU LOVED YOURSELF, WHAT WOULD YOU DO NOW?

- Do you take your tea breaks and do you eat a proper lunch at work?
- Do you work reasonable hours?
- Do you say yes when you long to say no?
- Do you go to the toilet when you need to?
- Do you make sure your needs are met?

Self-love at work is the same as anywhere else. Whether you're an employee or a business owner, if your needs at work aren't met, you won't feel taken care of. Your level of need at the end of your work day shows whether your needs were met during the day. Pay attention to how often you finish work feeling desperate to rest/ eat/ have time alone/ numb out with wine, video games or TV/ treat yourself to something you know isn't good for you ...

Have you ever stayed sitting on the uncomfortable chair, or delayed eating when you were really hungry, or remained at your computer even though your eyes were aching and your body felt stiff? At work, there are many small moments where your own needs seem secondary to the workplace's needs. But if you regularly override your needs at work, you'll eventually feel unhappy and dissatisfied (this applies to work as well as everywhere else). It's really simple: if you don't eat, listen to yourself, go to the toilet and rest when you need to and make sure you're treated with respect, you won't be OK.

EXERCISE: ASK YOURSELF THE LOVE QUESTION DAILY

Ask yourself the Love question daily—in relation to your eating habits, your hours or your relationships at work.
- If I loved myself, what would I eat for lunch today/ how would I organize lunch for myself daily?
- I know there's so much to do and no one else will leave before seven and it'll look bad if I do. If I loved myself, if I am precious to me, when and how would I choose to leave work today?

- If I loved myself, what would I choose to do now about my colleague's demeaning comment/ my boss shouting at me/ not being given the information I need?

If your work life includes challenging relationships and needing to stand up for yourself, make sure to read "In Your Self", which includes chapters on loving yourself in saying no, boundaries and relationships.

Now let's hear how some other people have dealt with challenging work situations. There are too many possible work scenarios for me to give an example of each, so see how you can adjust the ideas to your particular work situation and environment. I wonder whether any of these stories will resonate with you and how you'll love yourself differently after reading them. Let's start with Pauli's story.

Boss from hell

Like many people, Pauli feels he has a "boss from hell". A powerful and erratic man, this boss is making Pauli's life miserable: "One moment he's my biggest buddy, talking me up in front of my colleagues, and the next he insults me in front of everyone or blames me for errors he's made himself!" Pauli is highly stressed by this treatment, but he treasures the job and loves his work: "If it wasn't for him being my boss, I'd be so happy there."
With so many friends and family advising him to leave, Pauli feels torn. So he's sought counsel.

After discussing the situation, I ask Pauli to pose our Love question: "If I loved myself, what would I choose to do now?"

IF YOU LOVED YOURSELF, WHAT WOULD YOU DO NOW?

To his own great surprise, Pauli's answer is, "I would stay exactly where I am. This boss is helping me learn to tolerate someone being angry at me and not to take it personally. He's helping me learn to feel safe." I can see it's his Truth because his face lights up, a smile dawns and he suddenly seems energised and hopeful—very different from a few minutes ago.

When I prod him further, Pauli tells me his powerful father was an alcoholic who was extremely erratic: loving one moment, and shouting at and hitting Pauli the next. Pauli had anxiously tried to please his father to keep him in a good mood. As a boy he'd always blamed himself for getting things 'wrong' and his self-confidence had been badly affected.

After his enlightening realisation about the similarities between his relationship with his father and his boss, Pauli feels energised: "I've always wondered what it would have been like if I'd understood as a child that my father's outbursts were because of his own issues, and not because of me. Now I have the chance to try it out!"

As Pauli returns to work, he feels optimistic about this longed-for opportunity to heal an old wound. His boss remains erratic, but Pauli handles it better, and over time he no longer feels stressed by it. When he eventually moves on from that workplace, it's with a glowing referral from his boss.

So your Truth can surprise you and take you places you couldn't have imagined. You just need to ask your Heart for guidance. Thando's journey is a great illustration of this.

Radical listening to yourself

Thando is a free-thinking, constantly moving guy—commitment is tricky for him, and he flinches at anything that restricts him. He spent his early life being strongly moulded to conform to others' expectations, first by strict parents and then by an equally strict all-boys school. Now in his late twenties he's learned to conform, but it's crushing him: he is full of self-doubt and struggling to find his authentic voice.

New ideas and creating is what Thando does best, and one day a company approaches him wanting to implement an idea of his. They want him to be part of the creative team, but his fear of commitment makes this difficult for him. Finally he agrees to a short-term contract.

Learning to work with a supervisor and action his idea on a day-to-day basis is really challenging for Thando, who resists routine. It isn't just a matter of rebellion—his healthy need for independence and freedom was frustrated as a child, so he's protecting himself from feeling that way again: being told what to do every day feels like a death threat because as a boy he felt that he died a little inside.

Slowly but surely he becomes more involved and committed to the project. But every time the question of a renewed contract comes up, he becomes restless and anxious. Certain it's time to leave, he feels torn and confused.
In the therapy room, his answers to variations of the Love question surprise him: "I would choose to stay. I want to see how the project grows and be part of it."

So he agrees to a longer contract, and then another, and the choice to stay continues to feel safe and good because it's self-loving and is meeting his needs. It begins to surprise him how long he's worked on the team, but his need for independence has been met because this is his own choice. Even when things become difficult, he can look back and say, "I chose to be here, so let me see what else I can learn." Thus he figures out how to be his true Self.

Over time, he becomes restless and the contract renewal question emerges again. This time, when he poses the question, his self-loving answer is, "I want to do something new." Again this answer surprises him because the project has only just reached a point where he can coast a little after setting everything up.

"I think I like the setting-up part. I want to let someone else do the running-it part," he says reflectively. The Love question has shown him his Truth each time, which has given him a better understanding of himself and his deeper needs. As he's gotten to know himself, he's begun to doubt that Self less, and he's found that he loves the feeling of following his Truth. Any other way begins to seem untenable.

It's a strong and safe feeling when you act on your Truth—even if it's deeply challenging. When you've made a choice guided by your Truth, you can stop questioning the choice and just move forward—knowing it's your best path. Once you get a taste of this amazing feeling, you want nothing less.

Then things become even more interesting for Thando. He wants to learn more about himself, about what he wants to do next, about how to listen to and trust himself in every aspect of his life. He knows now that he definitely wants to leave his current workplace, but he doesn't know where he wants to go next.

Up comes the Love question again. He looks at me with wonder-filled eyes—which I've learned means the person has tuned into their Truth.
"I just want some time to *be*," he says. "I don't know what I want to do, but I don't feel it's really important right now. Something will come. For now, I want time for myself. To learn how to just be and feel."

It's a scary plan but it feels so attractive to him that he saves up, puts things in place and gives his notice. And then he goes home and does 'nothing', which meets his deep need for freedom and quiet. What he's actually doing is asking himself versions of the Love question non-stop, in both big and small ways.

"I'm practising Being and Doing," he tells me one day. "I am practising knowing deep within me when it's time for one, and when it's time for the other. I've noticed that it's a bit like breathing. You do one, and then you need to do the other. After you 'be', a desire to 'do' naturally rises up, and then after a while of being busy with 'doing', it naturally feels attractive to 'be' for a while."

Whenever he becomes anxious or doubts his choices, he checks in again and feels the very same Truth: *This is what I want to be doing right now*. Each time, this answer energises and reassures him, and most of the time he's happy.

"This is a formula for life," he tells me. "I hope I can remember this rhythm when I'm fully back at work. I want to live like this." After a while, work starts to gently flow in, ideas arise and wonderful coincidences show up—as they do when we tune in to what is right for us and act on it.

Practising the Love question helped Thando heal from the constant pressure he'd experienced in childhood to do what others wanted of him. During childhood, nobody really asked him what *he* needed. Now he's learned to ask himself. Thando is doing his best to listen to his own rhythm and act from that Truth, no matter what life brings his way. He's found out who he is, and let that Truth emerge into the life he's creating. He is amazed at how satisfied he feels.

Thando is self-employed; can you do this if you work in an organisation? Let's join Evelyn next as she struggles to follow her Truth while staying in a workplace she knows is bad for her.

Feeling powerless in the system

You may have noticed this from these last two stories:

We often find ourselves in—or, to be more provocative, create for ourselves—work situations that mimic dynamics from our childhood.

At work we interact daily with people who are each playing a unique role. Our first experience of that kind of set-up is in a family or at school—so it's not surprising that our emotional and psychological patterns from childhood can be triggered at work. In fact, this replay allows us to heal from and master developmental challenges we didn't manage to complete in our younger life. Basically, we get a do-over. Bosses typically symbolise parent figures or teachers, colleagues are like our siblings, cousins and school friends, and so we once more act out our inner dramas and wounding in this imaginary family or school. But this time we hope to find a love-based resolution and meet the needs that were not met back then.

The way our systems are designed to seek healing is marvelous, but if we aren't aware of this process and don't actively use it to heal and grow, it can feel like we're returning again and again to the same bad situations.

Healing occurs when we manage to truly love ourselves in contexts and situations that were pivotal in our learning to *not* love ourselves. It can take a number of attempts.

Evelyn comes to see me because she's feeling depressed. By nature she is vibrant and full of energy, but at this point her zest for life is low and she isn't sure she can go on.

In my line of work I hear a lot of tragic stories, but I sit and gaze almost open-mouthed as this beautiful, competent, sassy woman tells me the shocking story of her childhood, during which she experienced violence, molestation and abuse. Some members of her family perpetrated the abuse, while others ignored it and expected her to just get on with her life. To survive, she's learned to put on a believably positive front, regardless of the pain inside. It's hard to believe this has happened to her as she seems so OK.

When Evelyn starts to speak about her workplace, the dynamics of her childhood immediately become apparent. For several years she's worked in assisting and supporting children, a mission that resonates deeply with her. The organisation, she says warmly, feels "like a family". Then she shifts gears and says that she feels abused by her bosses, powerless in the emotionally unsafe atmosphere and that things are unequal among the staff.

I think: *No wonder it feels like family to her!*

Her response to her work situation is similar to her response to her childhood situation: she fluctuates between outrage and depression, rebellion and submission. She hides herself amongst other employees, who also feel disempowered. They're like children complaining about their parents' behavior but powerless to do anything about it.

Without realising it, Evelyn has returned to her role as the abused child, doing what she's learned to do: pretend that all is well, despite the fear and depression she feels inside. This time, thankfully, her Self is not going to play along. Her needs have been unmet for too long, and depression has now made it impossible for her to hide her feelings from herself. It's helping her become conscious of her situation.

"What is your dream?" I ask. "What would you love to do?"
"I'd love to leave and work for myself, but I'm too small. I can't go out on my own." She looks so convincingly adult when she says this that I have to listen closely to realize how much she sounds like a young child.

Over many months we work on the Truths that are becoming clear to her—about her family, her relationships, her work, herself—and she stays at the same organisation. She takes breaks from our sessions for months at a time and then schedules an appointment because things are bad again. Each time we talk, she gains new insights, new strengths, yet while she makes great strides in speaking out, looking after herself and not taking on other people's projections, she can't break the chains and leave her job. Random things keep happening to her that she feels are little nudges. She worries that the negativity at work will make her ill.

One January day I ask her, "If you loved yourself, what would you do now?"
"I'd leave," she says. It's been the same Truth each time. Then, sounding like a little girl, she adds, "I'd get myself out of this bad, awful situation." Her eyes light up, her face shines and she giggles at the feeling that comes with that Truth.
"What can you do to leave?" I ask, feeling the need to get practical.

She immediately shifts back into her familiar feeling of powerlessness and frustration, and I recognize that we are playing out her inner dynamics: she gets frustrated, pushes to make a change, feels the excitement of potential freedom and then shuts it down by returning to feeling small and powerless. I want to introduce something new.

"What would it feel like," I ask, "if you made a solid decision to leave. To look after yourself and take yourself out of this 'bad, awful' situation?"
"Oh, it would feel so marvelous. Free and exciting," she sings out joyfully.

"Is that something you really want? Does it make your heart sing?" I ask.
"Yes! Definitely," she answers without hesitation.
"So, if you decided to leave, what would you need to set in place to be able to do that?"
"Well, I'd need to save money. I wouldn't want to feel scared about funds. And I'd maybe need to start taking a bit of part-time work to build up my independent practice. Also, I have all sorts of ideas about things I'd like to do." She is back in her adult self, confident and capable.
"What would it feel like," I want to know, "if you decided to leave at the end of this year, and use the rest of the year to prepare for that?"
"Oh, that's plenty of time," she says. "It would get me focused and excited."

I want her to feel the contrast of the two options available to her so I ask, "How would it feel if you did *not* make that choice to leave?"
Her face crumples and her shoulders droop. "Oh, just dreadful. I become depressed just at the thought." She's silent for a minute. Finally she says quietly, "I can see what I need to do".

"So, if you loved yourself, what would you choose to do?" I ask again, feeling a little like an evangelical preacher.
She answers with enough oomph to please any preacher. "I would get myself the hell out of that bad, awful place and look after myself. I'm capable of it, so I'm going to do it!"

After that she pops in sporadically for sessions and to work on her issues, but she never again mentions the plan to leave work. Then she lands up in hospital with an infection.
"Another wake-up call," she texts me.
In my reply, I gently allude to our session where she'd faced the choice to stay or leave work.
"There is no choice," she texts back. "I'm leaving."

More health issues arise. As far as I know, she hasn't left yet, and that's OK. She's slowly putting things in place to be financially independent, she's learning more about herself. One way or another, she'll make choices that will meet her deeper needs and bring her to what she most longs for—even if her body has to push her to do it.

Evelyn's story is important for various reasons. One is that it helps to highlight how difficult it can be to act on what we know is our Truth. Another is that knowing our Truth and slowly working our way towards living it *is* already a loving choice. Sometimes just listening to and acknowledging our own Truth is the most loving choice available. The journey of life is not about 'getting it right' or reaching a desired outcome. Once you get to where you want to go, a new desire emerges anyway, so you may as well relax into the journey itself.

Sometimes we need to live outside our Truth to understand it better.

Sometimes being unloving is the way we learn to appreciate love. There's no textbook right or wrong way to live and learn. It may seem as though Evelyn is not managing to overcome this huge hurdle, but in fact she is unwavering on her Truth journey: trying, learning and communicating with herself is self-love and it's something she's had to learn from scratch. Taking the actions you know will meet your needs is not always easy—especially when your needs were ignored in your childhood, as hers were. As she keeps asking the Love question at every little choice, she will feel increasingly good about herself regardless of whether the outcome looks 'right' or not—or how quickly she gets there. Just asking herself what she needs already meets the need to be treated with care and respect.

The question isn't, "Am I getting it right and does it look good to others?" It's "Am I loving myself with what I am choosing right now? Is it meeting my deeper needs?"

There are many reasons it might be difficult to follow our own Truth. Dean in our next story, for example, is worried he'll let his employees down if he follows his Truth.

If you loved yourself, what kind words might you say to yourself about your choices so far?

 Pause now, take a breath and say something loving to yourself

When following your dreams feels like betrayal

"I've received a solid offer to buy my company!" Dean tells me one day in our session.
"This is what you've been working towards. Congratulations!" I say enthusiastically and then, when he doesn't respond in kind, I ask, "But why do you look distressed?"
"Well," he replies, "it's great for me, but I don't know what'll happen to the twenty people I employ. They've got families and lives. One is supposed to retire next year ... We've been like a family all these years. We're being bought out by a huge international organisation—my business will be incorporated into one section of it. It's a small asset that will streamline a process for them. For them it's a business deal—it's not 'important' in any personal way. They don't have close relationships with their staff. I don't know if I'll have to retrench any of my people. I don't know if I can face that. I don't know what to do."

Dean and I look at each other; our faces mirror each other's pain and concern about this serious situation. I know how long this man has wanted to change careers, and selling his company will allow him to follow his dreams. But I also know he won't do it at other people's cost.

I've used the Love question long enough to know that it's always the person facing the dilemma who will know the most satisfying solution.

Dean takes a moment to frame his situation and then asks, "If I loved myself, what would I choose to do now?" A moment or two passes as he allows himself to hear and feel his response. Then he slowly says, "If I loved myself, I'd stop worrying. I know this is definitely what I want. If I carry on in that workplace after I've had this chance to get out, I'll become very unhappy. So that's not even an option. What I know for sure is I'll do everything in my power, as this unfolds, to make sure all my employees have a safe landing. This change needs to happen, and I can't protect people by sacrificing myself. First, I'll get more information in writing from the new company so I know exactly what my employees are facing. Second, I'll make sure they get offered fair working conditions at the new place. Third, if they choose to leave, I'll use my contacts to find them other jobs. And I'll give them good leave packages so they have a running start. This might even push people into making their own changes they've been wanting. I'll have an interview with each one individually to see where they are in their lives and if I can maybe help them follow their dreams too. It won't be easy—I know that. But if I look out for them in this way, I'll be more at peace about leaving." He looks sad and thoughtful but no longer distressed.

"How do you feel about it now?" I ask gently.

He sighs. "Well, I'm quite nervous to deal with their reactions and fear. But I feel more ready. I know I'll be true to myself and to them. I think I felt like I was betraying them and everything would be lost—the relationships and trust we've built over the years—but I see now this is something we have to figure out together, like we always do. There's a small part of me that's a bit curious about what each person will choose and what I can organize for them." He lifts his head and I see a small smile emerging. "And there's a little part of me starting to feel the joy and excitement about my dreams coming true."

In the next story, Valan faces real financial consequences if she doesn't follow her Truth. But will she be able to stand up for herself?

Feeling abused and disrespected

A well-respected PhD in her field, Valan is involved in setting up a project for an international organisation. This thriving project has the potential to save millions of lives, and she has put all her drive, passion and intelligence into it. She's overcome huge hurdles of funding as well as people's resistance to change and reluctance to take responsibility, but she has been undeterred and now it's happening.

The only problem is that she's been hired on a short-term contract. Over time, it becomes clear that the project's magnitude has been seriously underestimated so that when her contract ends, the project is nowhere near completion. The organisation asks her to stay on, but doesn't finalize a new contract. Each time she raises the subject, she's told that funds are tight, and while she receives no definitive answer, she assumes it will be sorted out. She's so busy with the project that she brushes it off and keeps working.

Time passes and she becomes increasingly worried and upset at this treatment. She now hasn't been paid for months of work, but she doesn't feel she can walk away because the whole thing will collapse—and the project is aimed at helping many disempowered communities. She feels trapped and disrespected, and isn't sure what to do. Her friends and family are outraged at her treatment.

Valan is extremely talented and competent but she often doubts herself and avoids confrontation. As her superiors fail to acknowledge or financially reward her input, her fears and doubts about herself are being realized. As we so often do, she's manifesting her inner fears in her environment. This is useful to our growth because it helps us see these often-hidden beliefs better so we can make more self-loving choices.

Finally she reaches breaking point. Deeply upset and disheartened, she decides she has to walk away. As important as her beloved project is, she can no longer sacrifice her well-being for it.

'Hitting the wall' like this is usually a very powerful time of choice: Because the old way hasn't worked, we're pushed to let go of some illusion we've been holding on to, and so we find the courage to act. Ironically, our 'last resort' is often the time we open to our deeper Truth. It's a pity to leave this trick until we're experiencing real difficulty. It is instead possible to learn to let go faster and turn inwards for answers sooner, which is far more efficient—and a lot less painful.

A choice between a 'want' and a 'should' is a huge gift of self-discovery. Valan 'wants' to stay but she can see that in order to preserve her self-respect, and emotional and financial well-being she 'should' walk away.

She asks herself the question: "If I loved myself, *really* loved myself, what would I choose to do now?" And in that vulnerable moment, with all options open and available (as opposed to what she's been rigidly hanging on to), she suddenly sees a surprising third option that will benefit everyone.

The very next day she contacts those involved and shares her idea, which includes a way she can be paid for her work through a third party. Everyone agrees, and the project moves on in a way that works better than before. Valan does leave the project a while later, but by then her work is done—both on the project, and on herself.

Doubting ourselves makes things so much harder. In the next section I share an incident where I really had to trust myself.

Learning to not doubt yourself

A large part of this journey of listening to yourself is learning not to doubt yourself, because judgment and doubt block love. ("In Your Self" explains more about fear and judgment.)

Sometimes the guidance from your Truth feels so far outside of your norm that it's scary to act on it—but not acting on it feels even worse.

Here's an example of a stretch I needed to manage in a work situation where my Truth was contrary to my logic.

I was setting dates for a workshop I was running. My sister was coming to visit from overseas and said that she'd love to attend. Her interest and engagement felt good to me, so I set the dates to coincide with her visit. Then I heard that two people who had expressly asked to come couldn't make the dates I'd advertised. I was so disappointed. I don't run this workshop very often, and I wanted them to be able to attend.

I felt torn: on the one hand I had two very interested paying customers; on the other there was my sister (who had offered to pay, but that wasn't part of my consideration). Logic told me I should change the dates to accommodate two people over one—and for more money besides—but it didn't feel simple or easy, and I felt stressed by the decision. Some need of mine was not being met, but I didn't know what.

IF YOU LOVED YOURSELF, WHAT WOULD YOU DO NOW?

So, as I do in all times of confusion, I turned to my own wisdom, my Truth. I brought my dilemma to mind and asked, "If I loved myself, what would I choose to do now?" Then I felt it out—this date versus that date.

I was surprised by what happened. When I thought of my sister attending the workshop, I was filled with warmth and my heart opened joyfully. The other option felt fine, logical, good for business—but nothing like the happiness that arose with the alternative. I went back and forth a few times picturing each scenario, and there it was again: joyful happiness when I thought of one; cool, rational practicality when I thought of the other. Both were fine, but the more delicious option was meeting a need.

Doing this exercise reminded me that the main motivation in my work has never been money. I enjoy money and am happy to receive it, but I do what I do because I love it. I relish the excitement and feel honored to watch and support others' growing and healing, and I do it for the growth and learning I gain for myself.

My Truth turned out to be the illogical choice: if I loved myself, I'd choose to accommodate one person who would pay a reduced fee over two who would pay full price. It wasn't at all what I'd expected, yet it was the obvious choice once I'd seen it, and I experienced a deep remembering of my Self. I still didn't know exactly what need was being met by my sister attending, but it felt good.

You'd think, after that process, I would feel solid in my decision, right? But I didn't. I felt less stress, but stress was still there. I was afraid and I continued to question it: *But am I sure it's the right thing to do?* Each time I thought of the people who couldn't attend the workshop or felt stressed about the dates again, I reminded myself of my happy Truth feeling at the privilege of having my sister there. I'd remember, *This is what I chose*, and settle back into trusting myself.

The extra gift was that this Truth choice pushed me further into intimacy—with myself and my sister—and stretched me to practise not second-guessing my Truth even when it seems the less logical thing to do. It wasn't exactly comfortable, but it felt much more exciting than doing the workshop for business's sake. I had a tingle of glee and anticipation each time I thought about it.

In the end, the workshop was very special and the combination of people was just right. It probably would have worked out well whichever way I chose, but it was the experience that was most important for me—of respecting my needs and feelings, even if I couldn't explain them rationally. One way simply felt more honest, more meaningful and more true than the other. It would have been so easy to override that subtle Truth, but I didn't. I still feel proud of that now.

Is there a dilemma you're facing in which you're doubting yourself? If you didn't doubt yourself, how would you feel about the options available to you?

If you loved yourself, what would you choose to do now?

CHECK IN

How do you feel about your work right now compared with at the start of this chapter? Has anything changed in how you view your needs and your workplace? Say something kind about your work right now. Then keep reading. Try to do this a few times throughout this chapter. By the end you and your work may have a new relationship.

In our next story, Aiden doubted his Truth at his workplace—with unhappy consequences.

He throws himself 'under the bus'

Very often we feel that our problems at work are the fault of the workplace.

We often blame our unhappiness and unmet needs on the system, colleagues, bosses, unfair labor practices or low pay.

If these factors are contributing to our unhappiness they definitely need to be addressed, but working in a difficult workplace gives us the opportunity to improve our ability to self-love. Asking the Love question will help us step out of the quagmire.

When Aiden did this, he realized some very profound things about himself.

"I've been subpoenaed to testify in a case against a work colleague," he tells me in anguish. When I ask if he'd been aware of his colleague's wrongdoing, he answers, "Yes, I knew, but what she was doing was no worse than what a lot of our bosses are doing." He tells me how, a while back, someone had reported on a colleague and it had been the whistle-blower who'd been fired. "He was fired because he called attention to things that management weren't dealing with. Why would I put myself at risk by speaking out?" It turns out that the last two people who were asked to testify in this sort of situation had lost their jobs.

"So, are you worried you'll be fired?" I ask.
"I'm not actually," he says after some thought. "I have too much dirt on them for them to want to mess with me. I've cleaned up their messes too many times. They won't fire me." He looks proud and defensive as he says this—which is interesting given that he's just spoken with distaste and judgment about those very messes.
"What do you mean 'cleaned up their messes'?" I inquire.
"They've ordered me to cover up things they've done. I didn't want to, and I

told them, but it was my job and I had to—more than once."

Aiden is a proud guy who experiences chronic back problems. Knowing this, I ask, "How did you feel about having to bend over backwards like that?"
"I hated it."

We begin to explore his work situation and how he feels about having to compromise himself. It's a very uncomfortable conversation for Aiden because he knows he's doing something outside his integrity; he fluctuates between feeling bad about himself and saying how terrible his workplace is.
"So why are you still there?" I ask.
"I guess I'm scared to leave. I don't believe in myself enough."

So we look at his fears and desires about leaving this company: "I won't get such a good salary again ... I'm not qualified enough for other positions ... I have it good there ..."
After listening to a few of these reasons I softly ask him, "What is the price on your integrity and well-being?"

For a long while he looks at me in silence and then quietly says, "I need to leave."
"What would you do if you could leave?" I ask.
Suddenly he brightens up and out pour a whole lot of exciting plans. They are realistic plans, and we discuss the pros and cons and practicalities. Towards the end of our session, I ask, "If you loved yourself, what would you choose to do now?"
"I would begin to set my dream in motion and slowly make plans to leave," he says with a smile on his face.

When Aiden allowed himself to be compromised at work, he chose not to love himself or meet his needs. He blamed all of his unhappiness and unmet needs on his workplace: "*They* don't care about the human being in the job.

They compromise my integrity. *They* are willing to throw me under the bus to save their own hides. For *them*, it's all about the money." Yet he was staying in that position for the money, at the cost of the human being in the job—which was *him*! By doing things that left him feeling ashamed and disconnected from his Truth and well-being, he was throwing *himself* 'under the bus'.

These reflections are very uncomfortable for Aiden. He was so sure his negative feelings are because of his environment. But when he realizes that liberation and self-empowerment can come from taking responsibility for his own needs, he gets excited. *Really* excited.

I write the Love question on a piece of paper and hand it to him. "This is a high-speed connection cable to your Truth," I tell him. "Check in with it at every decision point."

He gazes at it the way someone looks at a winning lottery ticket. "This is exactly what I wanted!" he says joyously.

Aiden is still on his journey of learning to look within for the love he needs instead of feeling constantly hurt and disappointed that his environment doesn't respect and value him enough. His backbone is getting stronger. He has to get even better at seeing what his needs are and making choices that will meet them. In time, as he loves himself more and more, an environment that treats him in an unloving way will become impossible for him. He simply won't accept not having his needs met.

Do you love yourself at work? How does your environment treat you?

Is your environment reflecting something about the way you treat yourself?

This applies as much to employer as it does to employee as you'll see in

Serena's struggle.

If you loved yourself, what would you choose to do now?

Why can't they see it from my perspective?

Serena doesn't look at all serene as she enters my therapy room—she's riled up and needing to vent.

"I'm so annoyed," she tells me. "I know exactly what I want but they keep messing it up." She's talking about the design team working on her new product. "It's like they just can't see the bigger picture. Everyone's so concerned about protecting themselves and not looking bad that they don't communicate, and then they blame each other when things go wrong. Instead of the team I want, it becomes a finger-pointing contest and I'm like the mom disciplining children. I hate it! Why can't they just take responsibility? And because they're so touchy, I feel bad correcting their work even when they don't do it how I want. But I have to give feedback because I'm holding the vision—it has to be exactly the right color and exactly the right approach otherwise it's not *my* product." She takes a breath. "I've tried to let go and let other people have more say but then their choices aren't in line with my vision. There's often nothing wrong with what they choose, it's just not what I'd choose—although sometimes I'm shocked just how much they don't get what I'm trying to do. Why can't anyone else see it? When I do it myself, they're impressed and love it and it works, but when I try to help them they feel belittled by my comments."

I sit and listen to her frustration. Serena is a fast-moving innovator and I'm not surprised others are left confused in her wake. I'm also aware that she can be impatient and her style of communicating is sometimes abrupt. Serena needs things to be efficient and of high quality, and she often feels misunderstood and alone. She means well, but I can imagine what her employees say behind her back.

"I feel trapped. If I do it myself or get involved in their work, two things happen. One is that I look controlling and uptight—which makes me feel horrible. Two is that instead of appreciating that my way works so much better, they get upset and offended. I hate that moment! They cross their arms and I can see they've withdrawn, while all I want is collaboration. I want them to be open and enthusiastic to create together. Why can't they take what I suggest and add their skills to it, correct me like I correct them and then work together for the best outcome? Why do I have to be 'the boss' and they have to resent me? It's like I'm the only one who cares if this business succeeds. That's all I want, and it'll serve them too, but they just don't see it. I just want to be a team with them, but I'm excluded."

It's not easy to be the one with the vision leading others who don't see it. Many innovative leaders feel this—it's the classic 'lonely at the top' experience. In some work environments, we compare ourselves and are afraid of being 'less than' others. This kind of insecurity blocks the possibility of opening up to real engagement and collaboration because people are constantly afraid of losing face and being wrong. Just like in sex (see Chapter 8), where if you're constantly worrying how your body looks naked, you can't relax into the experience of physical connection, if you want to create in a satisfying way, you have to accept yourself and allow yourself to be just the way you are. Serena mostly accepts herself, but because she really wants her team to like her, she holds herself back in a way that leaves her feeling frustrated and rejected—and that's when her communication becomes sharp and shaming, which exacerbates the distance between her and her employees.

"If you loved yourself, what would you say to yourself now?" I ask.

Serena groans and rolls her eyes at me. The Love question irritates her—she finds it easier to look for the cause in the other people and 'fix' them. But our sessions have helped her and she's learned to trust my strange ways, so she gives the question some thought.

"If I loved myself ... I would say to myself ..." She's lost in her inner world for some time and then suddenly snaps to attention. "If I loved myself, I'd allow myself to be me. I'd stop apologising for myself. I saw an interview with a woman once and she said, 'I will not apologize for my excellence'. I like that. I'm good; I hold the vision for this. If they can't see that, it's not my responsibility. I can't feel bad about my role as leader."

She looks calmer, but I also see the familiar blame-game—that this is other people's fault. I want to help her ease her relationship and communication style.

"That's a good start," I say, "but it leaves the other people on the outside. If you loved yourself, what would you choose to do about connecting with them?"

Again she rolls her eyes—other people are not her favorite thing. "Well, if I *have* to ... If I loved myself ... I'd see that it's not really about me. They're challenged and for some reason they're scared by what I show them. I mustn't take that personally. I know when I get frustrated, I say things they get angry about." She notices my piercing look. "OK, OK, I also wouldn't like it if someone spoke to me that way." Then she looks down and says softly. "I feel hurt when they pull away from me, so I want to hurt them back. I know it's my defence."

Catching this rare vulnerable moment, I ask Serena softly, "So if you loved yourself, what would you choose to do now?"

"I'd like to learn how to talk to my team in a way that they listen and don't pull away from me."

"What do you think might help with this?" I ask quietly.

"*You're* the professional! Aren't you supposed to tell *me* that?" she demands, annoyed.

I smile. I understand she feels exposed right now and is covering it with anger and blame. I reflect this to her.

"Ugh! Fine!" she exclaims. "If I loved myself, I'd say nice, *kind* things to myself and to my team mates." She's getting there but she still doesn't see her role in the dynamic.

"Do you think you treat them as your team, who're on *your* side, or as people who need to do what you tell them?" I enquire.

"Well, I *want* them to be my team … as long as they're the way *I* want them to be a team." She smiles ruefully, seeing the irony.

"If you approach them in that way, where they're separate from you and can get it wrong, how safe is it for them to relax and be innovative and connect with you as a team?" I ask.

"But it's not all my fault!" she bursts out. "I've given them so many chances, you have no idea! I've *learned* to feel this way. I *want* to work together with them."

"But do you see them as equals?" I persist. "Do you value each person for their unique gifts and skills? Do you appreciate both their abilities and their limitations? Do you express your appreciation?"

"I *have* tried that," she says morosely. "I'm not a total idiot. I know I need to affirm people. But they just can't do stuff the way I wish they would. I just don't know what else to do. That's why I come to *you*." Her sarcasm tells me she's defending herself from difficult feelings.

I ask how she's feeling right now, and she wails that she's feeling alone and misunderstood, just like she feels with her employees. "What would make you feel more seen and connected with me right now?" I ask gently.

"If *you* at least got it."

"So, is it up to me to make you feel seen and understood?" I want to know. "If you loved yourself, what would you say to yourself now?"

"Well, if I loved myself—which I *don't* feel right now, by the way—I'd say to myself that … I actually know you get it more than most. Maybe because I talk to you about how it feels to me. And I know you don't *mean* to leave me alone ... and ... maybe if I talked a bit more about my feelings rather than getting sarcastic and angry like you show me I do, then people might be less scared of me." She sits quietly in thought. "Maybe I could try to be more open and relaxed with them ..." She looks up at me and sighs. "This is going to take a lot of practise."

For the first time in this session, we both feel a glimmer of hope for the change she longs for.

How do *you* defend yourself when you feel exposed and vulnerable at work? What are the outcomes of this choice?

If you loved yourself, what would you choose to do now?

 Pause now, take a breath and say something loving to yourself

And *your* workplace?

Serena's learning is true for all of us.

As you become more self-loving and follow your Truth above all, you'll find that either the environment begins to shift and treat you differently, or that you will very easily and organically move to one that better reflects the consideration and care you offer yourself.

If your situation at work is not flowing or you feel things are out of balance, ask yourself the Love question. Open up, listen carefully and be prepared to be surprised, because the answer might not be what you expect. Remember, if it is your Truth, you'll feel it expanding your chest and lightening your heart. You will *know*. That's because your needs will be met by the answer and that feels good. Then do your best to follow it—even if at first it's only by acknowledging that it is *your* Truth.

It can take time to be ready to take your steps. Money, family and other considerations may mean you need to go slowly.

Be gentle with yourself and honor your situation.

Keep asking the Love question and listening. Your path—and the right timing for you—will reveal itself as you go along.

Following your Truth can be exciting: you may find yourself having serendipitous meetings and events, and you never know what will come up. When it's your Truth you're following, your needs are met and your heart feels happier so you feel safer and more open to life, other people, love ...

Life at work can be just as satisfying as your 'off' time.

Work is something you are doing. It's part of your life experience. For it to be a deeply satisfying daily experience, you need to stay aware of your basic and deeper needs and dedicate yourself to respecting them as best you can *while at work*. Treat yourself with respect. Look after yourself. Make sure you eat properly, go to the bathroom as needed, work the hours and the way that honors your needs. Strive to not compromise your Truth by agreeing to things that feel uncomfortable or painful to you. Take it step by step. Ask yourself the Love question, listen to yourself and follow the Truth that emerges ... at your own pace. Are you ready to feel satisfied and loved at work?

If you loved yourself, what would you choose to do at work now?

END OF CHAPTER CHECK IN

- What are your views on meeting your needs at work now?
- Have they changed in any way through reading this chapter?
- What would you like to say to yourself about loving yourself at work?
- Is there any decision you'd like to make now about you and your work?

Do the meditation video again and read the chapter summary to help you clarify your views and intentions. Write down your intention for yourself at work—you can use the chapter summary to write on.

Here's the one-page summary of this chapter to download now and remind yourself of the key points of loving yourself at work.

DOWNLOAD Chapter 4 summary
www.ifilovedmyself.com/members/chapter-4

Chapter 5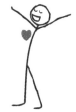

If I loved myself in my Body and Health

Under the sustaining influence of love, the physical body is always at its best. It is probably true that more people are sick from lack of love in their lives than from all other causes put together.
Eric Butterworth

SET AN INTENTION FOR THIS CHAPTER NOW

Setting an intention is a way to add power to something you are doing. Your intention is about your own needs and desired outcomes; it's unique to you and where you are in your life right now. Examples might be:
- My intention while reading this chapter is to understand what my body is telling me
- I have the intention to love and value my body more
- I intend to learn how to meet my needs so that my health improves.

 Before you work through the chapter, scan this code to join me for a short video meditation about setting an intention for yourself and your body.

You can also access the meditation through this link:
www.ifilovedmyself.com/members/chapter-5

Learn the hidden language of the body

Your body is an essential part of you, so it makes sense that if you love yourself, you will also love your body. But for many of us, loving ourselves is itself a massively complex issue, and we're definitely not always pleased with the body we have.

We may dislike our shape, skin, face or height. We sometimes resent or fear how our body functions: our body may have a disability or be inclined to obesity or illness. Society gives a big thumbs-up to healthy, capable and aesthetically shaped bodies. If we happen to have a body like that, it's easier to feel empowered and free to love our body than if we have one that triggers society's fear or rejection. Having a socially disapproved of body—in terms of aesthetics, ability or health—can make a person feel trapped and disadvantaged. It's more challenging to appreciate that body.

Your body, like you, thrives in an environment of love but declines when there is a lack of love.

No matter how you feel about your body—love it, hate it or something in between—you cannot live on Earth without it, so some level of peace is required. One way to start appreciating it is to understand how it helps you love yourself.

Your body is a good friend who wants the best for you.

Your body is a sensitive indicator and reflects in minute detail which of your thoughts and behaviors is low on love and if your needs are not being met. Emotional, physical and behavioral symptoms are the language your body uses to communicate with you. I love the metaphor of our needs being like a child needing the toilet. If you don't listen when she announces that she needs the toilet, she'll wait a while and then tell you more urgently. If you silence or ignore her, her call will get stronger, louder and more distressed. She'll pull at you, act out and finally, if you still don't attend to her need, she will mess on the floor. And you'll have to clean it up. Sometimes a symptom seems to come out of the blue but often a symptom or illness results from not listening to, or acting on, what you need and often by the time you're cleaning up the mess, you've ignored a message for quite a while—like in these situations:

- You feel tired but you don't rest. You push yourself to do too much and don't set boundaries to ease your load. You feel increasingly tired and irritable, and eventually you get a bad cold.
- A woman looks after everyone else. She puts others' needs ahead of her own, even if it means she goes without. She's wonderful and nurturing and generous to everyone else, but inside she's hungry to feel cared for too. One day a lump is found in her breast.
- A man is very stressed at work. He's afraid of losing his job and doesn't speak out about the injustices he sees there. He tells his wife he's starting to feel like a pressure cooker. At home, he shouts at his children. He begins to get headaches that cause blurry vision. His doctor tells him he has developed high blood pressure.
- A student has to do a presentation. She's terrified of speaking in public and fears she might pass out or die during the presentation. On the morning of the presentation she wakes up with laryngitis.

Our body talks to us all the time. Even expected symptoms—such as the body's reactions to chemotherapy or pregnancy—are your body communicating with you. If you listen well, then like the child who needs the toilet and is taken in time, it will often respond with gentler symptoms that pass sooner.

This *does not* mean it's 'your fault' if you get sick.

Having a physical problem—or even dying from a disease—

does not mean you've failed or are getting something 'wrong'.

Weirdly, sometimes becoming ill or having a disability greatly enhances our optimal development. It's just a way your body helps you develop your Self or change patterns that are not fully self-loving. For example, when your resources are low, you're pushed into setting the boundaries you tend to overlook when you have enough resources not to feel the impact of doing the things you don't want to do. When someone starts a project or business, has a new baby, gets a serious illness or finds themselves tight on money, they suddenly have to look after themselves more carefully just to be OK. Then when that nosy neighbor comes over to chat (again), or the energy-draining friend asks for money (again), or the school committee asks you to run the fair (again), your situation forces you to finally say no when you have never had the courage to do so before. In other words, your decreased capacity helps you do something you couldn't manage before.

Having an illness or disability and facing death or preparing to die can help people ask for help, open up to intimacy or express their Truth for the first time in their lives. It can make people listen to themselves more carefully, nurture themselves more or learn things about themselves they were unaware of. There are many ways our body's dysfunction can support our journey towards loving ourselves more.

This is by no means easy—especially if your challenge is life-long or severe. The body is a stringent teacher of self-love, but its methods can be powerful, for example:

- When we're very demanding and critical of ourselves, being physically unable to do things offers us an opportunity to learn to be kinder to ourselves.
- When our body can't do things other bodies can do, it helps us look for our

worth beyond 'being useful' or 'normal'.
- When we use an activity to avoid dealing with things in our lives, being unable to do that activity pushes us to listen to ourselves differently.
- When we've been afraid to speak our Truth, put ourselves out there and shine, having a serious illness forces us to face death as a reality and make different choices in life.
- When we're frightened of and judge our own needs, being dependent and unable to meet them can help us learn to love and accept ourselves and our needs.
- When we're uncomfortable with intimacy, needing others to help us physically pushes us to open more to others.

Illness, pain and physical disability—major or minor—can be difficult but wonder-filled teachers on the journey to self-love. Since your body will continue to teach you until you part ways, consider taking this approach:

Your dis-eases and disabilities are helping you master or become an expert in something.

Ask yourself, "What is this experience helping me to master?" and, "How can I undertake this learning in the most self-loving way?"

Your body communicates with feelings, energy and health.

Whenever your body expresses any kind of pain, discomfort or weakness, it's a call to stop, look and listen.

Increased good feelings, energy and health are a thumbs-up, indicating that your needs are being sufficiently met. Anything else suggests that you are ready for the next level of self-care. Whether you have a minor tummy ache, a chronic condition or a syndrome that presents itself regularly, you can gain a closer and more fulfilling connection with yourself by viewing your symptoms as loving messages from your caring body, who just wants you to love yourself well.

There are tips throughout this chapter and specific exercises at the end to help you learn how to ask your body what it's saying and how to listen to its responses. What is your body lovingly expressing to you right now with its symptoms?

If you loved yourself, what would you say to your body now?

 Pause now, take a breath and say something loving to yourself

Imagine decorating your worst flaws

I sit opposite my beautiful friend and enjoy looking at her as we catch up after a long time. Her face sparkles with new piercings that enhance rather than detract from her beauty, and when she tells me her story, I understand why.

During the time we haven't seen each other she went through a series of painful experiences and rejections that left her wondering if something was wrong with her. She went to therapy and looked at the things in herself she's always felt bad about, and this time, instead of beating herself up about them, she decided to take brilliant positive action.

"Here," she says excitedly, pointing lovingly to one piercing. "I had a dent from a really bad pimple when I was fifteen. I always felt self-conscious about it, so I decided to decorate it. And this one makes me aware of how I wipe my nose—I have to do it with care. I can't just smash a tissue over it like

I used to. And this one makes me aware of how I put things over my lips. I'm more aware of what I put in my mouth now—we don't realize how rough we are with our faces."

As she speaks I can feel her joyful appreciation for these reminders to be mindful. I appreciate the sparkle of her jewels and wonder how rough I am with my own face as I wash, clean, pick and wipe it.

Then she continues her show and tell, raising her sleeve proudly. "I used to hate my arms. I have this rough skin here, so I never showed them." She uncovers a matrix of cubes tattooed on her upper arm. It looks to me like dragon scales made of sacred geometry—delicate and magical. It obviously does have healing power because she goes on to say, "Now I want to show my arms! The pain of the piercings also did something for me. It grounded me into my body in a different way. It made me realize I am here right now. I carry that with me too."

I sit there amazed at how she's managed to find such creative ways to love the things she didn't like about herself—that she judged not good enough and that blocked her from loving her body. I wish everyone could hear what she's saying.

"Can I put your story in my Body chapter?" I ask, and she laughs delightedly in response.

So here she is. I hope you gain something from witnessing her bravery.

If you loved yourself, what would you choose to do about the parts of your body you judge as 'not enough'?

Are you laughing often enough for your health?

Remember the adage, 'Laughter is the best medicine'? Well, it's true. More and more research is showing that the chemicals, proteins and hormones released by your body when you feel joy, love and gratitude are the most effective treatment for any and all physical and mental disorders. It seems that if you want to be healthy, your best bet is to frequently wallow in good feelings. Sometimes it helps to know a bit of the science behind such claims, so I'll briefly explain the link between our emotions and our physical state. I hope by the end of this you'll throw yourself with abandon into laughing and enjoying life, and the next time you see a child having fun, encourage him to do it *even more*, instead of curbing his joy because you're worried he'll mess up the lounge ...

Our emotions play an important role in making sure our needs are met—they are the first messengers. (This is explained more in "In Your Self") If we ignore our feelings, our subconscious mind needs to find another way to get its message across. And the second messenger is the body.

The body uses symptoms to alert us to the fact that our needs are being ignored. All mammals show physical symptoms when they experience an out-of-balance emotional state. This is because every thought or feeling triggers the release of tiny chemical proteins called neuropeptides (NPs). Every emotional state has its own distinguishable and measurable frequency. The frequency of a specific emotion galvanizes photons within your cells and throughout your neural pathways to release appropriate NPs—for example, hormones, endorphins, cortisol and adrenalin—which in turn play a critical role in metabolic function.

Positive emotions stimulate beneficial NPs such as endorphins or oxytocin.

These are the 'feel-good' chemicals we seek through exercise, laughing, chocolate or lovemaking. Negative emotions prompt the stress chemicals connected to our 'fight or flight' response, which help us respond or take immediate action. These stress chemicals are fun on a roller coaster or bungee jump, but if they are continually released over a period of time they can hinder rather than help your body. That is how stress diseases like ulcers and high blood pressure come into being.

EFFECTS OF EMOTIONAL STATES

Science is now able to demonstrate the physiological effects of emotional states. According to scientists, a protracted negative mental state predictably weakens your body, and a positive mental state strengthens it.

EMOTIONAL STATES THAT WEAKEN YOUR PHYSICAL SYSTEM BECAUSE OF THEIR LOWER VIBRATIONS	EMOTIONAL STATES THAT STRENGTHEN YOUR PHYSICAL SYSTEM BECAUSE OF THEIR HIGHER VIBRATIONS
Shame	Trust
Guilt	Gratitude
Apathy	Appreciation
Grief	Optimism
Fear	Willingness
Anxiety	Acceptance
Anger	Forgiveness
Hate	Understanding
Resentment	Love
Hopelessness	Reverence
Jealousy	Joy
	Serenity
	Enlightenment

Thankfully, physical symptoms tend to only emerge after we've held a certain emotional state for quite some time.

Our physical symptoms reflect our deeper patterns of thinking and feeling.

Once set in place, the 'chemical programming' of our body is quite persistent—familiar thoughts and behaviors repeat the same chemical responses. Changing a pattern we have 'switched on' requires that we purposefully 'reset' it. Even if you've changed your lifestyle and situation, the underlying chemical and thought patterns can remain—like a default program.

The good news is that in every moment, each of us has the power to raise our vibration and change our state of health. Instead of waiting for your body to call your attention with pain or health issues, or ignoring your body when it does so, you can actively choose to increase your beneficial neuropeptides.

How?

Love yourself more. Laugh a lot. Listen to your Truth and act on it. Listen to your body. Meet your needs constantly. Appreciate things. Languish in good feelings when you have them. Spend your life in prolonged states of gratitude, trust and love.

Ask yourself often, "If I loved myself, what would I choose to do now?" And then do it.

The next sections explain how disease forms and how self-love can help prevent illness.

Do you know what your body is saying?

When we love someone, it's natural that we care about their welfare and do our best to listen to what they tell us. Think of a person or a pet you love—you genuinely want to know what he or she is communicating because it matters to you.

You'd think we would also do this for our body because obviously it matters to us—a lot! Without it, we couldn't live. But many of us have weird relationships with our bodies. There are many ways our body communicates to us—and even more ways we avoid listening. The thing is, many of the things our body tries to tell us are not convenient for us to hear. In a capitalist, productivity-driven society, the need to rest or slow down is a threat to our success. 'Success' might mean anything from earning money and fame to parenting, meditating, improving your mosaic technique or running faster around the block. Our society teaches us that more, faster and newer equals 'better'. Our bodies don't work according to this principle, which is often inconvenient.

A glaring example of how our society views this inconvenience is in advertising. A commercial will show people overindulging in foods or doing activities that strain the body. When a character's stomach becomes acidic and uncomfortable, he or she will take an antacid: problem solved. Another character will develop a stress headache, so they take a painkiller: problem solved. Someone's body will be tired, so they'll receive a vitamin B injection: problem solved. Inflammation? Muscle pain? Use this cream: problem solved.

But is it really?

I'm not against pain relief or medication—I'm grateful for the alleviation of pain and the healing it offers. It's just that I would much rather see the guy eating that fast food/ stressing himself at work/ overexerting at the gym choose things that feel better to him. What makes me shake my head sadly is how commercials reflect our society's tendency to ignore our bodies' messages. Especially when these *inconveniently* tell us that something we're doing is not meeting our real needs.

We need to learn our body's language. Why? Because it shows us the path to our Truth and joy. What is this language? Let's see.

Your body's wisdom

Earlier in the chapter we touched on how our thoughts and feelings impact on good or poor health. Now I want to explain how our repeated patterns of thinking and feeling lead to specific ailments.

Recent research in the fields of neuroscience, psychoneuroimmunology, neuroplasticity, neurobiology, quantum physics, epigenetics and nutrition is showing very clearly how our thoughts, feelings and lifestyle affect the illnesses, discomfort or health we experience in our bodies and minds. More and more books and articles are informing us that we have a lot more influence on our health and well-being than we previously imagined. A lot of this influence begins in the brain, so let's start there.

Your brain's primary task is to help you stay alive. To this end, it constantly scans the environment for threats to your survival. Information flows into your brain through your senses, and once the brain recognizes a pattern, it informs your body to take the action that kept you alive the last time you encountered that same pattern. In other words, your brain is like a super-computer—every split second, vast quantities of data are processed and commands sent out. Most of the time we're completely oblivious to this—to be conscious of it would be overwhelming.

The brain gives commands by sending electrical impulses down neural pathways. Like little messengers, these impulses trigger the appropriate parts of the body to release chemicals, hormones and proteins that will create the desired actions—anything from spiking anxiety to help you escape a situation, to telling you to ignore a droning noise so you can concentrate on your exam, to pushing you to give that little bit extra in the gym. Everything you do—from a flinch to a blink to a squat—is ordered by your brain.

Feelings and emotions are part of this system. Feelings make us move towards or away from things: fear or pain makes us avoid, pleasure makes us approach. Feelings are therefore very useful tools for our brains in guiding us to survive.

Most of us live quite repetitive lives. We have the same routines, live in the same places, see the same people. We also have many of the same thoughts every day. As we repeatedly meet the same stimuli, so the same neural pathways and the same areas of our bodies are flooded with the same chemicals, proteins and hormones, over and over again. One might anticipate that there would be some wear and tear in the 'high-traffic areas'—and that is precisely what happens. If you, for example, keep having the same worries and your brain sends out the same stress messages, your body will repeatedly produce the same relevant chemicals to cope. As this happens over and over, your body slowly begins to develop 'stress symptoms'—high blood pressure, indigestion, ulcer, etc. Those symptoms are the result of 'wear and tear'.

Your body reflects your thought and emotion patterns.

If we were to flip this, we could surmize that someone with hypertension, indigestion and an ulcer is likely to be having regular stress-inducing thoughts about something that causes them pain and anger (ulcer), that they find difficult to digest (indigestion) and that is limiting the free flow of joy (hypertension) in their lives. From a psychosomatic perspective, you begin to get a picture of someone's deepest issues simply by knowing what ails their body.

Your body doesn't lie and it's not 'out to get you'. It merely reflects your patterns, and so offers a beautiful opportunity to learn to listen to yourself. Your body is communicating with you—and if someone we love is communicating with us, we want to listen, right?

In the face of society's teachings to ignore our body's wisdom, paying attention to our own body in an honest way requires intention and effort. The counsel of your body may go against what you perceive to be 'good for success': "What do you mean, I need to rest?" we demand of our overstretched, caffeinated, sleep-deprived body—"I need to keep going if I want to get this done." This is not rational: studies show that insufficient sleep has a negative effect on productivity, planning, organizational skills and creativity, *and* it makes you more prone to weight gain. So a stress-bunny who never stops moving yet who's nevertheless overweight might, ironically, need to sit down and rest to shed those kilograms. Any time you attend to your body's needs, it will function more efficiently.

So here we have it again—if you don't listen to your Truth, you can't meet your real needs and you therefore won't function optimally or have consistent well-being. Next time you have an ache or illness, ask yourself the Love question: "If I loved myself, what would I choose to do now?" I'm not promising that you'll like what you hear or that it will be convenient, but it will always be better for you in the long run. Like any other area in your life, as you follow your Truth, the path to resolving your physical issues will become clearer.

To summarize this massive topic: your body reflects your thought and emotion patterns. So what is your body saying to you? What are your deeper needs at this time?

CHECK IN

How do you feel about your body right now compared with at the start of this chapter? Has anything changed in how you view your body? Say something kind to your body right now. Then keep reading. Try to do this a few times throughout this chapter. By the end you and your body may have become better friends.

When Lisa, in the next story, listened to her cancer, she heard some powerful messages.

If I loved myself, what would I choose to do now?

Cancer can be a friendly message

By the time I met Lisa, she'd spent the better part of five years undergoing intrusive and taxing investigations, operations, treatments, chemo and radiation therapies for various cancer-related issues. Side effects and unintended consequences of each intervention had left her riddled with nausea, aches and body parts that didn't work as they were supposed to. Each time we met, Lisa's body was expressing something—ranging from mild discomfort to intense pain.

It didn't occur to her to talk to me about these things. She was so used to them that she'd accepted them as part of the physical journey. She'd come to talk about her emotions and how to cope in her life. When at first she mentioned some pain or another and I asked about it, she shifted into reporting mode. Well-trained by the medical world, she would list her physical experiences in a monotone, academic sort of voice. I could see this list of symptoms was what her many doctors required of her, but it wasn't what I was seeking. Even though every one of her many symptoms had a legitimate medical cause, I wanted to find out why her body was expressing its discomfort with that particular symptom at that particular time.

If her neck was hurting, for example, I would ask her to give me the first expression or idiom she could think of that used the word 'neck.'
"A pain in the neck," she might say.
Then I'd ask, "What is a pain in your neck right now?" And out would pour whatever was troubling her most painfully at that moment. Always at the end of the conversation, I would ask, "How does your neck feel now?" and each time she would test it and look at me with huge eyes and say, "It feels much better now! I'm amazed. I never knew my body was talking to me like this!"

Given how medically legitimate each of her physical complaints was, even I was amazed at what emerged from Lisa's symptoms. Each time we asked, traumas and old memories stored by her body emerged for healing and clearing. The connections and meanings of her symptoms were astounding—and very much related to her illness.

Slowly, her body became an active participant in our sessions. We would talk to one body part and it would ease but another part would suddenly hurt or make itself felt because it had something to add.

One day she confessed, "I realize now that my body has been telling me the same thing for years. I knew what I needed to do the first time I got cancer. I knew how I needed to live my life. I did it for a while, then stopped. When I got sick again, I realized the same thing, but I didn't do it. I don't know why. But this time I *have* to focus on doing it. I need to live my life for me and not be afraid anymore."

Nowadays, I'm happy to say, Lisa is in full remission. She has learned to see her body as a friend, not an enemy. While she still frequently forgets, she does her best to listen very closely to its messages, rather than try to 'fix' it. That way, she finds she can meet her real needs better and her symptoms pass sooner and more gently.

The idioms and metaphors we use daily show that we've always known the body expresses our emotional and cognitive habits. We say someone 'bends over backwards', 'sticks her neck out', 'doesn't have a backbone', 'is a thorn in our side', 'doesn't have a leg to stand on' and 'feels sick to their stomach' …

Here's one technique I use to help access messages from the body.

EXERCISE: CRACKING THE CODE OF YOUR SYMPTOMS

1. Think of a body part or symptom that is bothering you.
2. Without giving it much thought, bring to mind an idiom or expression about that body part. Don't judge, analyze or try to change what emerges. Just notice the first one that comes to your mind.
3. Now ask yourself, "What does that expression mean to me? How would I explain it to someone?" Don't try to find the 'correct' answer like for a test. The important thing is what it means to you.
4. Once you feel clear about its meaning for you, ask yourself, "How is that relevant to me and my life right now? Is there anywhere or anyone with which I am doing this thing?" Use your idiom, for example:
   - "Where am I bending over backwards right now?"
   - "How am I biting the hand that feeds me?"
   - "How am I carrying the weight of the world on my shoulders?"
   - "Am I sticking my neck out anywhere?"
5. Trust the first answers that pop up.
6. Now that you know what this symptom is reflecting to you, you can choose what to do about it—how to love yourself more in that place. Ask, "If I loved myself, what would I choose to do in this situation now?"

If no answer comes to your question about your idiom (step 4), don't stress. Say to your body, "I am open to hearing what you have to tell me. Please show me in a way I will understand." Then let it go—it'll come. Or perhaps one of the other exercises at the end of this chapter will suit you better.

Get to know (and love) your enemy

The other day during meditation this thought popped into my mind: "I should be *so* grateful for the parts of my body that have been causing me pain and discomfort." Out of the blue, I suddenly felt a deep sense of joyful appreciation for the exact parts of my body I sometimes worry about, consider dragging off to the doctor to be 'fixed' or fear to be signs of some serious degenerative disease ... Love for *those* parts! Really??

It's because *those* parts of my body are taking me on a journey. They are my guides to my Self, of course. They're guiding me home to me. To Love.

How do you start to love something you really wish wasn't there—like pain, illness or disability? How can you love what scares you? These are Big Questions.

Viewing symptoms as communications from yourself to help you love yourself more can bring some relief—or at least some curiosity. In a way, your body is like a child. Children—including our inner child—are excellent indicators of balance and imbalance. When your (real or inner) child is acting out, doing things that drive you mad or you cannot understand, assume he or she is trying to communicate that something is out of balance. Some urgent need is not being met, and they need you to attend to it. (For more on children, see

Chapter 9, "If I loved myself in my parenting".) Your open, non-judgmental listening can help bring him or her back to healing balance. The difficult-to-love behavior is merely a sign that the child is feeling disconnected from Love. Really and truly, that's all it is. Trust me, I'm a psychologist.

To reconnect to Love, your body needs your help—listen and open your heart to your body as best you can. I want to add here again that having physical symptoms doesn't mean you don't love yourself, or you're getting something 'wrong'. It's sometimes just a way you're being offered to learn another level of love—love in difficult spaces.

If you're someone who was born with a physical challenge, the task you're faced with is to love yourself with your aches, pains and disabilities and do all you can to ease their effects while living your life as you and loving all of who you are—exactly as you are. No apologies.

What are your experiences helping you master? How do your challenges push you to live your Truth more? How can you love yourself better because of your body's journey? Lorna's story on page 124 is an illustration of this challenging journey.

When your body behaves in an unusual and uncomfortable way, it's merely lovingly reflecting that something you do regularly is detrimental to you. How can you find out what that is? Sit down in a quiet space and open your heart as best you can (one way to do this is to become aware of the center of your chest and imagine it softening and gently warming and opening like a flower. It can help to think of something you find cute—like a cuddly puppy or someone you love or something you feel grateful for). Then holding that feeling, talk to the part of your body that's in discomfort. Chat to it. Say hi. Ask it how it is. Ask if it has something to tell you. Ask if there's anything you could do that would improve the discomfort.

Listen to the answers that arise within. Don't judge or question them. Just receive them as your inner Self communicating with you.

Neuroscience tells us that the way we can begin to accept—and even love—our enemy is to start getting to know them better. When you stop judging or trying to control and instead seek to communicate and understand, you find that all anyone ever wants is love and peace in the form of acceptance, respect and harmony. This is also true for your body. Try to open non-judgmental lines of communication with things that trouble you, and see what happens.

When I did this with my shoulder that had been hurting, I received a surprising response. Here's what happened:

Just ask your friendly body

I ask myself, "Hey, painful shoulder, what needs are you showing me? If I loved myself, what would I choose to do now?" and my shoulder instantly answers, "You'd give yourself a break."

When I say 'answers', I don't mean I hear a little voice, but more that I get the words and meaning in my mind—like a thought—and I can feel the feelings that come with it. I stay still and open to hearing what else my shoulder has to say.
"What does that mean?" I ask it. (Yes, you can have entire conversations with your body parts!)
Immediately I perceive the message: "Don't be so hard on yourself. Don't put yourself down. Lighten up and it will lighten your load." As I stay open and listening, it continues: "You seem to think you have to carry it all. But trust life more and let others decide for you a bit more. Walk lighter and

with more ease. Then I won't have to stand frozen and tight in an attitude of preparedness for the big burden that's always about to land on me."

Whew. That's quite a message.

Excuse me for a bit—I need to take a few moments to digest this. I feel somewhat tearful. I'll be back in a few minutes ...

*

OK, I'm back. This message isn't new to me. I know I have this tendency and I also know that I've manifested pain in my shoulder *because* I have this repeated pattern of thinking and feeling that's not fully self-loving.

In order to help me listen to my Truth and begin to lovingly meet my needs, my shoulder has started to express louder (i.e., more painfully) so that it'll be harder for me to ignore. It hopes I will stop and listen. Hearing the message now, I feel loved. I hope I remember it. But if I don't, my shoulder will no doubt kindly remind me.

Like training wheels on a bicycle, pain tends to persist until we no longer need its help.

It's not easy to change who you are and how you habitually think. I've been working on this particular fear-based pattern of thinking for a long time, and it's much less, but still there. In time I hope it won't be.

It is possible to alter these thought patterns though, and that's particularly necessary if your goal is to transform a physical symptom. You change by loving yourself more. You change by choosing your actions from a place of self-love and so better meeting your needs. While the change is sometimes quick and easy, other times it can take years to slowly shift your patterns of thinking—and this is especially so if they're connected to how you thought you would survive in the world as a child.

Author Louise Hay was publishing books about the connection between dis-eases and patterns of thought as early as the 1980s. Years ago, when I first encountered her famous little blue book, *Heal Your Body*, I followed her suggestion: I wrote a list of all the physical problems I'd ever had and then used her book to look up the thought pattern and recommended affirmation for each one.

I was somewhat skeptical when I saw that all the thought patterns and affirmations for my list were variations of the same thing. "Ha!" I scoffed. "She writes the same thing for everything! Pah. 'I love myself this, I love myself that, I trust the Universe ...'" It felt like those fake fortune tellers who tell everyone, "You will meet a tall, dark stranger and go on a journey."

Then it occurred to me to look up some ailment I'd never had ... and guess what? The thought pattern and affirmation were completely different to the ones on my list. At that moment I realized that all the physical symptoms I'd ever had were different expressions of the same patterns of thought. This is the reason my shoulder's message is not new to me. I recognize it deeply.

Your body holds your highest Truth, indicating when you're not honoring your real needs. Stepping away from your Truth is not self-loving. In my case, my shoulder is telling me that it hurts me to believe I'm unsafe. My Truth is to relax, let go and trust. Doing that meets my deeper needs, so I feel good. It leads to my best health and most joyous life—and my physical symptoms ease or disappear. I've experienced it, witnessed it and read about many more people who have released their physical symptoms this way.

I return to my main message in this book:

When we don't follow what our greater Self already knows, we do not love ourselves. Not really. When we love ourselves, we live in line with our Truth. We listen to our needs and meet them.

If you don't feel good in some way, you're simply out of sync with your Truth. If you want to know what your Truth is, just ask the part of your body (or the symptom) that's holding the indicator: "Hey, Body, if I loved myself, what would I choose to do now?"

Listen to what it tells you. Then start doing it. No step is too small if it's in the direction of your Truth. Rory's story below is a great example of this.

It's OK

Rory is in terrible physical pain just before her big presentation. She keeps saying how upset she is: "I'm so pathetic to have manifested this now. I should be enjoying this moment and yet here I am, incapacitated. I just can't let myself have the good stuff I create. I'm so angry with myself. And it really hurts!"

It's painful to listen to her being so unkind to herself.

I venture to ask her the Love question, unsure as to whether she can even hear it in this moment of self-flagellation, but surprisingly she does. She asks me to explain a bit more and then she's quiet for a while, thinking. Then she speaks: "If I loved myself, I would tell myself, 'It's OK.'"

Her answer seems so short and simple I'm not sure she's understood the concept, but then she adds, "It's OK that I got hurt at this time. It's OK. I'm not bad or stupid. It's just where I am right now. It's my pattern. I'm working on it. It's OK. I'm OK."

Being kind to yourself when your body isn't functioning the way you wish can be really hard. Here's Lorna's inspiring story of finding her way through a degenerative condition.

Loving yourself through unremitting disease

Lorna was diagnosed with a genetic degenerative muscle disorder when she was nineteen, just as she was preparing to fly from the nest. She's now thirty-three, in a wheelchair, and has watched all her friends create lives for themselves—lives like the one she dreamed of too. Hers now entails constant operations, physiotherapy, physical braces, large quantities of medications and regular emergency visits to the hospital.

"Look, I want to love myself, I really do," she says, "but I feel so angry about being stuck in this while others get to live and play. My body is such a disappointment. I really got a dud."

In exploring the Love question she finds she can appreciate and love herself for who she is and how she handles everything, but she just can't manage to love this body that's let her down so badly. "It's betrayed me", she says angrily. "It doesn't deserve my love or forgiveness!"

To tell her that her symptoms are a message from herself or to imply that she should just listen to her body more would be insulting. Lorna's body experience is extremely difficult but she's tired of being at war with it. Now she wants to find love and peace with all parts of herself, even her wretched body. She needs to figure out what to do differently in this situation to achieve that.

"I wish I could feel less angry. I wish I could feel less scared. I wish I was OK with this somehow – but how do you make peace with this? How do I accept that my body is going to slowly stop working and abandon me?"

Deep within one of these conversations one day, she asks herself the Love question again. For some reason, on this particular day, she's able to muster deep compassion for herself and finds herself answering, "If I loved myself, I would be my own best friend. I would encourage myself and believe in myself and never leave my side and always be the one with something good to say to me. It would be easier to deal with all this if I had someone like that with me, who I didn't feel I was burdening or fear that they'd had enough of my boring story."

She considers what being her own best friend would involve, and realizes that she's felt judged and abandoned by herself at times: "This is the body I have. I can't help it. And then it's like part of me has judged it as deficient and turned away from me. Like I'm embarrassed to be me, to have this body and this condition, and I don't want anything to do with me. But it's me! I can't avoid being with me. So I judge and feel repulsed by me and at the same time I feel hurt and abandoned—by me! It's crazy."

She likes this new idea of becoming her best friend. Over the next while she begins a period of reconciliation between the parts of herself. Many internal conversations and mediations are held. Slowly a truce begins to form, and she starts to take charge of her own experience in a different way. She speaks encouragingly to herself, she actively seeks out things that will strengthen her inner journey, and finds the work of Dr Joe Dispenza and Abraham Hicks very helpful.

"It's strange," she says. "Nothing outside has changed. My body is the same,

I still do the treatments and everything, but it feels different to me, easier to accept somehow, and I fight it less, and that makes it feel like less bad stuff is happening to me."

While it remains a daily journey, Lorna has reached her goal of finding some kind of peace within this experience. And she has her best friend doing it with her.

Does your body scare you?

I think body stuff is part of what's hardest about being human. Our body is our partner and guide on this journey, but we get angry at our bodies for scaring us. We feel like they can control us and we try to get power over them—it's all so complicated ... Yet it's simply a relationship, and like any relationship it needs to be regularly nurtured.

Nurture your relationship with your body.

If you're having a tough time with your body right now, give you and your body some couple therapy. Open up a compassionate reconciliation conversation between it and yourself. I hope you can accept and forgive how your body is different from how your head thinks it 'should' be and that you can open to the gifts it's offering you.

Regularly appreciating your body will help you and your body create a loving, caring partnership. Here's how:

IF I LOVED MYSELF IN MY BODY AND HEALTH

EXERCISE: **HOW TO FEEL JOY IN YOUR BODY**

The ability to sense and feel are the great delights of being alive—and you need your body for that. Think of something you love to eat. Think of how your lips, teeth, tongue, gums, throat and saliva glands all collaborate to give you the experience of a food's taste and texture. Think of when your eyes see something beautiful and how that translates into meaning in your brain and good feelings in your body. Think of when you're touching and being touched by someone you love, and how all the cells in your skin sing and vibrate.

Become aware of sitting right here right now, feeling fabric on your skin, air on your face and a chair or mattress against your body, breathing in and out, hearing sounds, seeing and smelling things … all your senses actively engaged. Pause your reading for a moment to feel all this and appreciate it. Allow this moment to seduce you entirely.

Allow life to seduce you all the time.

Regularly lean in to the joy of having a feeling, sensing body. Think lingeringly of people you love, and notice the pleasant sensations in your chest. Feel the air on your skin and surrender to it …

No matter how your body looks or how well it functions, it's a spectacular vehicle, the most complex technology you'll ever own. The things it can do! How it takes air into the lungs through the airways, absorbing just the oxygen into the bloodstream to be delivered through our blood vessels to every part that needs it. Amazing! The metabolic processes breaking down whatever rubbish we throw into our stomach. Genius! And the healing—oh my goodness, don't get me started on its incredible capacity for healing! It can repair itself magically!

Thank you body

Take some moments now to think of yourself and your miraculous body, and appreciate all it does and all it gifts you with daily. Tell it you love it.

"Thank you, dear Body, for being my home. Thank you for supporting me and doing your very best for me. Thank you for all the amazing things you do. Thank you for digesting and moving and pulsing and renewing. Thank you for all the things you feel and process. Thank you for the patience you show me as I do my best for you. I love you, Body. You are wonderful, and you are mine. I'm so glad we have each other."

> **DOWNLOAD** Thank you body
> www.ifilovedmyself.com/members/chapter-5

On the next few pages are three practical exercises to hear the messages from your body.

How to decipher your body's messages

Many of us will pay a lot of money for specialists to tell us how to correct the imbalances in our systems. Funnily enough, this information is readily available if only we choose to listen.

Your body is a storehouse of the patterns of thinking and behavior that don't meet your deep needs and so cause you to feel unloved and out of balance. You can simply ask for this information, and use your body's magic as your guide to self-love and improved health. Here's how:

EXERCISE: HOW DO I LOVE MY BODY?

This is a very rich 'getting-to-know-yourself' experience, which will reveal your current relationship with each of your body parts. The more honest and less judgmental you are, the more you will learn.

1. Draw or print out an outline of a body—your body—on a piece of paper. It doesn't have to be a good sketch—it can even be a stick figure.
2. This exercise works best when you focus on each body part methodically—head to toes or toes to head. Starting with your head or your toes, think about each body part in turn and let yourself be honest with what you think of and how you perceive this part of your body.
3. Try not to analyze or judge what comes up. Simply turn your attention to that specific body part and then observe the stream of thoughts and feelings that arise in response. For example, "My head: the lump that sits on top of my neck. It feels heavy when I think about it, like it's hard to hold up. It puts pressure on me sitting at the top like that. I feel irritated and resentful of its weight. I don't even want to give it more attention now—I just want to turn away from it. My poor neck, having to hold up this heavy head, having to bend and twist all the time."

- Trust what comes through, even if it doesn't seem to make sense. (Would it surprise you, for example, if I told you the person above has migraines and neck problems?)

4. If a color, word, sentence or strong feeling comes up, notice it and write it down on your body map. If you feel numb, bored, angry or tearful, write that down—it might make sense to you later.
5. Once you've gone through your whole body, sit back and look at your piece of paper. Observe the general feel of your comments and perception of your body. Based on these, how would you define your current relationship with your body? This is important information: if you generally feel good about your connection with most of your body parts, you'll feel good. Most of us have at least one or two areas we feel less at peace with, if not downright judgmental and angry. The next exercise will explain how to begin communicating with your body parts.

EXERCISE: BODY MAP

1. Draw or print out an outline of a body—your body—on a piece of paper. It doesn't have to be a good sketch—it can even be a stick figure.
2. Circle or color in areas in which you know you have imbalances in any way—aches, pains, disease, etc.
3. Connect with each part of your body in turn, even the parts you haven't colored in. You can work through your body methodically—head to toes/toes to head—or engage intuitively with whichever body part feels most relevant. Greet each part and ask it the Love question: "Hello, Head. Please tell me, if I loved myself, what would I choose to do now?"
4. Listen to what each part has to say. Try your best to not judge or analyze the response, and remember that what seems nonsensical will sometimes become clear later. Write down on your body map exactly what you've heard. Ask any clarifying questions you have, and write down the answers you sense.

IF I LOVED MYSELF IN MY BODY AND HEALTH

5. When each body part feels complete, say thank you and move on to the next. Pay special attention to the colored-in or circled parts—they have extra-important information because they indicate where you're somehow not meeting some needs.
6. You now have a map of your current inner patterns and the Truth actions that will heal them.
7. If you choose, you can engage more deeply with specific body parts. This will give an in-depth understanding of the dynamic that particular part represents for you, and what gifts it holds. (The next exercise gives more guidance on how to do this.)

EXERCISE: HOW TO COMMUNICATE WITH YOUR BODY

This exercise is effective for going deeper and starting to change the more difficult dynamics you hold in your body.

1. Turn your attention to an area of your body that elicited some unpleasant or strong reactions in the above exercises. Greet it: for example, "Hello, Hip," or "Hello, Eyes."
2. Notice how that feels. Very often you'll notice an immediate reaction: it may feel as though you are being called for mediation with someone. You'll have feelings about it—fear, anger, discomfort, relief, excitement. Just observe your responses without reacting. You want information, not argument.
3. Now ask this body part, "What is it you need from me?" Try to use a kind tone.
4. Sit quietly and listen to the thoughts and feelings that arise in response to this question. Don't be afraid if it seems crazy to be talking to your body—listen and trust the conversation you imagine is taking place. Open up, allow information to come to you in whatever way it does, lean in to it, let yourself listen to the loving wisdom your body has to offer.
5. To end (or as a quick version that you can do daily), ask your body as a whole,

"What is it you need from me?" (A variation of this question would be, "If my body had something to say to me, what might that be?")

6. Just listen and trust the answer, the 'knowing' that arises in response. This is how your body communicates with you.

Remember, your body is your vehicle for living as a human on this earth. Ideally you want to be at peace and living harmoniously with it—whether or not it's functioning or looking 'perfect'.

We listen to those we love. Love your body by listening to it.

If I loved myself, what would I choose to do for my body now?

> **END OF CHAPTER CHECK IN**
>
> - What are your views on your body's symptoms now?
> - Have they changed in any way through reading this chapter?
> - What would you like to say to yourself about your body and health?
> - Is there any decision you'd like to make at this time about your relationship with your body?
>
> Watch the video again and read the chapter summary to help you clarify your views. Write down your intention for yourself and your body and health—perhaps on the chapter summary.

Here's a one-page summary of this chapter to download now to remind yourself of the key points of loving yourself in your body and health.

> **DOWNLOAD** Chapter 5 summary
> www.ifilovedmyself.com/members/chapter-5

Chapter 6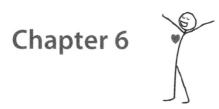

If I loved myself in my Food

One cannot think well, love well, sleep well, if one has not dined well.
Virginia Woolf

SET AN INTENTION FOR THIS CHAPTER NOW

Setting an intention is a powerful way of increasing the effectiveness of what you are doing. Your intention is about your own needs and desired outcomes; it's unique to you and where you are in your life right now. Examples might be:

- My intention while reading this chapter is to understand my patterns and the choices that don't serve me regarding food, and discover how I can do things differently.
- I have the intention to love and value myself with my eating choices.
- I intend to learn how to make peace with my eating and with food.

 Before you work through the chapter, scan this code to join me for a short video meditation about setting an intention for yourself and your food.

You can also access the meditation through this link:
www.ifilovedmyself.com/members/chapter-6

If I loved myself, what food would I choose to eat?

Ah, food—such a loaded topic for so many of us. There are many reasons we eat, and many ways food can be used to love or avoid ourselves. In this chapter I am *not* going to list which foods or how many calories are best for your body. Please kick all 'shoulds' out the room right now. My focus is on loving yourself and choosing food from your place of Truth. Your body *is* very likely to respond to this love with more vibrant health and balanced body weight—but more importantly, you'll feel loved. Ready? Here we go.

 Pause now, take a breath and say something kind to yourself

Aim for feeling loved in your food choices

Every bite you take reflects whether you're acting from a place of love and Truth in that moment.

The degree of joy and satisfaction you experience from eating something indicates how much you feel heard and loved by yourself—in other words, how much your needs are met by that choice.

Conditional food-love says, "I will only love you if you eat food I approve of." Conditional love sucks! It hurts to be 'loved' for what you do or have, rather than for who you are.

Instead of praising or shaming yourself for the food you choose to eat, aim to feel loved.

Ask: *Which food or drink will make me feel loved and cared for right now?* No one but you can say what that choice will be. Sometimes a greasy burger will bring a feeling of happiness and joy, and sometimes that feeling will come from a salad: it depends on your needs in that moment.

The food itself is less important than the feeling of being heard and loved by yourself. Your body is more likely to easily digest food that is eaten with joy than with misery.

The chemicals that flow through your system when you feel happy aid digestion and metabolism, whereas misery and fear inhibit optimum functioning.

Let's say you're comfort-eating and feeling miserable even as you eat. The unpleasant feeling reveals that something is off balance, that what you're doing isn't meeting your needs. The moment you become aware of your discomfort is the moment your true voice emerges from beneath the fifth slice of pizza. It might say, "I feel bad because I'm not listening to me. I don't feel loved or respected having this food shoved into me. I'm not even enjoying it."

It's a gift to notice when you're feeling unhappy or uncomfortable. Your discomfort alerts you to the fact that there's a choice to be made, and because you noticed it, you have the power to choose.

Ask yourself, "If I loved myself, what would I choose to do now?" Your answer may be, "I'd slow down and really enjoy what I'm eating," or, "I'd let myself cry," or, "I'd stop eating right now, wash my hands and go for a walk—and *not* shame myself for what I've just eaten."

Your Truth answer is always loving and will always seek to meet your real needs—the ones you were unsuccessfully trying to meet by eating all that food in the first place.

Your Truth is not conditional. Your lovability doesn't depend on what food you choose to eat.

Whatever your answer is, listen to it and follow your Truth right out of the pit.

If I loved myself, what would I choose to say to myself about what I recently ate?

What is healthy or unhealthy food?

When I speak about 'healthy' food in the context of loving yourself, I don't mean what the textbooks say is best for our bodies and minds. I mean the food that *feels* best to us: the choice that leaves us feeling strong and nourished and vital.

For example, I had a neighbor who was in her eighties. A mother of ten adult children, and granny to numerous grandchildren and great-grandchildren, she smoked like a chimney and ate a large—and I mean *large*—slab of chocolate every day. The *whole* bar. She happily chomped it up square by square throughout the day. It always made me smile to see that partially eaten slab next to her chair. She loved that chocolate—it was one of the things she lived for. To her, it was not 'unhealthy'. My guess is that daily chocolate bar did her more good than harm, because she was putting joyful emotions into her body.

The emotions you experience during and after eating your food are just as likely to impact your physical state as the material make-up of the food itself.

This is because your brain plays a big role in all body matters. Its main role is to keep you safe, so it's always on the lookout for danger. It informs your body whether food is safe to fully digest or not.

For example, you can eat a sweet cream pastry, enjoy it thoroughly, feel satisfied afterwards and think of it fondly for the rest of the day. From that your brain perceives that you are safe, and it floods your system with feel-good chemicals and hormones like endorphins and oxytocin, while lowering stress chemicals like cortisol. (See Chapter 5, "If I loved myself in my Body and Health" for more.) As a result, your body benefits—or at least is not negatively impacted—by eating that cream pastry.

Alternatively, if on eating the cream pastry you shame yourself for your lack of willpower and get frightened thinking of weight gain or how the ingredients will damage your system, your brain will perceive danger. It'll then flood your system with stress chemicals, proteins and hormones to prepare you for fight or flight. Your system then has to contend with a wash of adrenalin that has no outlet because there's no *real* danger to face. Metabolism and digestion are slowed by these chemicals, so your body struggles to deal with the cream pastry. You may think it's the pastry that has caused your indigestion or weight gain, when it may actually be your emotional interpretation: in this case, the negative impact of the sugar, dairy, fat and gluten might be negligible in comparison to the avalanche of chemicals that result from the emotional and cognitive interpretation of eating that food.

I do believe that if you choose to eat from a place of love, food can be 'healthy', no matter what it is. This is not permission to ignore your body: it does have preferences and will let you know if it's not happy with something you've eaten, and if you listen, you can choose differently next time. From a place of love. Listening to your Self is key to a healthy body—the next section explains how.

If you loved yourself, which food would you fully enjoy now?

How do I know what food is good for my body?

Your body gives you signals about whether a certain food makes it feel good or not. Learning what food makes your body happy is a matter of paying attention to how you feel after eating it: feeling light, energetic, even-tempered and vibrantly alive is an indication that your body likes what you've eaten; feeling bloated, sluggish, gassy, grumpy, achy or demoralized shows that your body does not prefer that food.

Each body will react to food in its own way. Some bodies prefer meat, starches or cooked food while others thrive best on raw greens. Some bodies can comfortably tolerate fried food, gluten, sugar, alcohol and dairy while others can't.

There's no food that's 'healthy' for everyone: you are unique, and you need to love yourself in your own individual way.

Follow your body's signals of health and well-being—you'll be amazed how self-loving it can feel to give your body the food it prefers and avoid the food it doesn't. It's not always easy to do though, as Susan's story illustrates.

If I loved myself, how would I listen to my body now?

You are what you eat

"Work lunch the other day was typical," Susan explains in a session. "Everything but the roast vegetables had wheat or dairy in it—and my body responds badly to wheat and dairy. The vegetables looked good, but when I'm really hungry I tend to eat food that I regret later. So I'm standing there, and what goes through my mind is: *Susan, if you choose the vegetables, you'll prove you can make responsible choices.* Because I *know* those vegetables are the right choice for me, yes? It's like, if I can eat the better-for-me option, I'll feel I have things under control. If I can do that, I'm OK as a person.

"But I look at the cheesy lasagna, and I'm hungry, and part of me really wants to just not care. What stops me going for it is that I'm also worried people will judge me for being fat and eating lasagna. So I've got this whole dialog going on in my head while I stand there deciding.

"And I *know* that lasagna—I've met it before. It leaves me feeling gross and gassy and unhappy. I know that, but I still want it. I also know my head will say to me afterwards: *Susan, you need to be more disciplined. You have no willpower. This just shows you can't handle responsibility. How are you going to get your life in order, be healthy, lose weight, get the relationship/ job/ life you want if this is how you behave?* All this going on inside my head makes me want to eat the lasagna *and* a big slice of the chocolate cake with cream they also have there, and just kill myself later."

You thought it was just about what to eat? It's not.

We sometimes interpret food-choice moments as a judgment on our worth. Why? To survive and thrive in any arena, we must figure out what helps us and what harms us. To do this, we constantly assess our environment. This useful and healthy survival reflex becomes problematic when we start attaching meaning and worth to something. Assessment turns into judgment when, instead of gauging things as 'good *for me*' or 'bad *for me*', we label things 'good' or 'bad'—and judgment blocks love.

How does this relate to food?

Like Susan, many of us judge ourselves and our worth by what we eat, and the dilemma of what to eat becomes one of: *How much do I love myself? How much do I think I'm worth?* Maybe we should turn a familiar phrase around and say, "You eat what you are." This partially explains why people who struggle to choose what to eat can end up flushed and distressed. Attaching value judgment to our food choices implies that we can get it 'wrong'—and none of us wants to 'get it wrong'.

Will I choose the fast-food and a carbonated drink, or the freshly made chicken and a fruit juice? could be rephrased as *Let's see if I'm worth loving based on the choice I make*. As we look over a menu or decide what to make for supper, the real question is not, *What shall I order/ cook?* but, *Do I love myself?* Ouch! This is conditional love at its nastiest and food guilt can hit hard—no wonder we crumble when faced with choosing between the fruit and the chocolate bar.

We must eat to meet our need for fuel, so it's really easy to assume we can eat to meet other needs like love or comfort too.

If you don't feel good after eating, you've probably been unhelpfully trying to meet *other* needs with food. The good news is that with food we can easily love ourselves more—just by checking in instead of blaming or shaming.

Even in the middle of a bite, you can ask, *If I loved myself, what would I choose to do right now?* Remember to connect with your heart as you do, and try to identify your real needs. Ask the Love question with genuine care for yourself, as you would to someone you really love. And be open to being surprised: sometimes the lasagna will be the most self-loving option, and sometimes it won't.

> **CHECK IN**
>
> How do you feel about you and food right now compared with at the start of this chapter? Has anything changed in how you view eating and food choice? Say something kind to yourself right now. Then keep reading. Try to do this a few times throughout this chapter. By the end you and food may have become closer friends.

How to know what you really want to eat?

Have you ever opened a restaurant menu and wailed, "I don't know what to order"? Choosing what to eat is a decision point. While it might be a small one, *every* decision point is a choice to love, honor and obey yourself—or not. This section gives clues as to why some people struggle to decide what to order from a menu—and hopefully some tools for making an easier and more satisfying choice.

Doubt in any form usually means we're trying to decide between what we *want* and what we think we 'should' choose. In other words, it's a choice between your Truth and what you think is the world's truth. The menu dilemma looks something like this: *I want* the spicy chicken wings [that you know will activate your heartburn] *but I should* have the grilled fish. We often rely on willpower to make the choice we 'know' is better for us. When our willpower fails, we later feel guilty. That's because willpower is short-lived. But listening to your Truth has staying power.

IF YOU LOVED YOURSELF, WHAT WOULD YOU DO NOW?

Henry looks at the menu and asks, "If I loved myself, what would I choose now?"

The fresh tomato-based vegetable spaghetti may seem like the obvious answer because he liked it last time, it's healthy and if he loved himself, he would put tasty, nourishing food into his body, right? Well, yes, but 'nourishing' comes in different forms on different days. Your mood, physical state, level of rest, body type, most recent meal and the time of the month all affect your body's needs and responses to food. While salad, for example, is usually viewed as healthy food, it's not always the 'better-for-you' option. The best option for you is based on the given moment, and only your body can tell you what that is.

So now what? How does Henry decide what to eat if he can't rely on what he thinks he 'should' order?

He must figure out his needs.

"Well, if I loved myself," he answers himself, "I would choose something satisfying and nourishing—something I enjoy and also feel good after eating. Let me figure out what that would be right now. Do I feel like something hot or cold? Hmmm ... I want something warm in my belly. OK. Do I want something light or something heavy? Heavy. OK. Salty, spicy, creamy, sweet? Savory, with a bit of richness. Something soft and mushy or something crunchy? Not mushy—I want something I can bite into. So that's not cold salad or soft pasta then. What else is on the menu? How about a burger? They make big, juicy ones here. Yum, yes! A burger is perfect. But I don't want chips—I don't want that heavy, greasy feeling. Salad instead? No, that would be cold and unsatisfying right now. How about warm vegetables? Yes!"

And there it is. Decision made: happy Self, happy tummy, happy body. Needs are met and Henry is feeling loved and nourished in all senses of the word.

It may sound onerous to have a whole conversation with yourself every time you sit down to eat. On the flipside, *everything* in your life, even one meal, is an opportunity to make yourself feel either listened to and cared for, or unimportant and a little bit empty. Does that still seem like just a small choice?

Are you ready to start choosing what you eat from a place of love and Truth? Let's review:

EXERCISE: WHAT DO I FEEL LIKE EATING?

Questions to help you decide:
I give myself permission to have any food I want. What will be satisfying to me right now and leave me feeling good?
1. Do I feel like eating something hot or cold?
2. Do I want something light or heavy?
3. Do I want a salty, spicy, creamy, sour or sweet taste?
4. Do I want a soft and mushy or firm or crunchy texture?
5. Which available option best meets all my chosen criteria?
6. Does it feel good to me?

_____

Put these questions on your fridge or in your kitchen to help you make love-based food choices.

DOWNLOAD What do I feel like eating?
www.ifilovedmyself.com/members/chapter-6

If I loved myself what would I choose to eat now?

What if I can't choose a self-loving food?

You don't always have access to the food that would meet your needs in any given moment—maybe there's very little food in the house, you can't get to the shops, you're at a catered conference or business meeting, or you just don't have the money for it. At such times, love yourself deliberately with the best option available.

Talk to yourself kindly as you make the next-best choice, and energize the food with love.

The 'make love to your food' exercise opposite might also help—although perhaps not at a business lunch!

Talking to your food

In many cultures it's the norm to sing blessings while preparing food or to pause before eating to express gratitude. This makes sense when you consider that this food will soon be incorporated into your system and become part of your body. How would you like to engage with the food you're about to merge with? Are you open to the pleasure of the union? Here's an exercise to practice savoring your body's union with the food you're eating.

EXERCISE: MAKE LOVE TO YOUR FOOD

This is a mindfulness exercise.

Greet your food. Be aware that you're about to bring it into your body. Take some time to really gaze at it. Notice the colors and textures.

Touch it, if appropriate. If it's a piece of fruit, gently rub it on your cheek and closed lips, noticing the sensations and textures.

Bring the food close to your nose and take a slow, deep sniff; savor the top and bottom aromatic notes.

Take a lick and focus on identifying the tastes and textures. Place a small piece of food slowly into your mouth, maybe rubbing it first over your teeth. Roll it around inside your mouth with your tongue. Slowly bite down on it. Notice the texture, the sound, the tastes.

As you swallow, welcome it into your being and thank it for nourishing your body.

Addictions

When people speak about being addicted to food, they usually mean that they use food to avoid dealing with something.

We have many socially acceptable ways to avoid ourselves and numb out—food is just one of these. I chose not to include a separate chapter on addiction because in a way this whole book is about treating addictions, be it alcohol, smoking, food, sex, drugs, work, TV, exercise, relationships, computer games, gambling, approval ... Sometimes we use food to hurt rather than love ourselves.

So, what is addiction? It's a dynamic in which you use something external to improve something internal—essentially your feelings. Addiction forms when you feel powerless to stop a regular behavior because you believe it's the only thing that will make you feel better.

The way to free yourself from any addiction dynamic is to allow yourself to feel the 'uncomfortable' feeling you're avoiding.

Instead of turning to something or someone else, learn to connect to yourself and turn inwards for support and love. (See 'How to feel your feelings' on page 36). Asking the Love question and listening to your Truth will reveal your unique steps to genuinely feeling better. When you do that, you meet your real needs, so you don't need to rely on anything outside to feel OK.

You are enough.

Connection is a vital part of healing from addiction so please get help from a professional counsellor, therapist, support group or someone you trust. Asking for help when you need it is a very powerful way of loving yourself and meeting your needs.

What things do *you* do when you feel lonely, anxious, sad, scared? Even if we're not addicted to food, we sometimes use it in unhelpful ways. The next section explains why.

If you loved yourself, what would you choose to do when you feel difficult feelings?

Why do we choose 'unhealthy' food?

There's a story I really like in the book *Zero Limits*. The author, Joe Vitale, tells how during a workshop he invited Dr Hew Len—a master practitioner of the Hawaiian healing technique *ho'oponopono*—out to eat, but there were only fast-food places around. He apologized profusely, but his apologies were brushed aside. They ate cheap burgers in a greasy diner and Dr Len thoroughly enjoyed his food. Afterwards he went to extend his compliments to the surprised 'chef' who had deep-fried his premade burger.

The health benefits of the food we eat may have less to do with what we put into our system than the energy with which we approach it. If we define 'healthy food' as 'whatever food feels best and leaves us feeling strong, nourished and vital in the moment', interesting questions arise: Why do we sometimes choose food that hurts rather than nourishes us? Why would we willingly choose not to love ourselves through food or other life choices?

In my private sessions, groups and workshops, I've noticed that themes of shame, doubt and self-hate often underlie our problems. Many of us walk around afraid that we're unlovable, not good enough and not important—though this is never true for any of us. The trickiest part of the menu choice is *not* the dilemma between healthy food versus tempting food; it's *not* a battle between Good and Evil. The real challenge is to know what's driving our choice: are we being motivated by self-love or by self-sabotage stemming from fear? When we make a food (or any other) choice from a place of fear or pain, we can unintentionally affirm the very thing we want least: *I feel bad, so I choose to eat this thing that will make me feel bad in the hopes that it will soothe my inner pain.*

Your painful feelings are there to show that you have unmet needs (More on this in "In Your Self"). If you're seeking to soothe an internal hurt, food is the wrong tool for the job—trying to distract yourself by eating will probably make you feel *less* loved. After a bout of what some call 'emotional eating,' we often shame ourselves: *How can I respect myself? Look at what I do!* This can create a cycle of feeling unloved, eating, feeling worthless, eating, feeling unloved, eating… All the while our real needs for feeling connected, affirmed and cherished, for example, remain unmet.

What if we used this cycle to our benefit instead? "Fake it till you make it" is a saying from the cognitive-behavioral stream of psychology—it means that if you want to behave and feel a certain way, sometimes the best approach is to just start doing it. Slowly that behavior will become more natural and more comfortable until one day it will be true for you.

You can practise choosing your food *as though you already love yourself.*

After a while, choosing those foods will make you feel better about yourself, and loving food choices will become easier and easier to make. It becomes true because by paying attention to and taking care of yourself you're already meeting your real needs.

That strategy is not always enough though. Addictions—to food and anything else—are complex. Ask yourself the Love question at every food decision point: "If I loved myself, what would I choose now?" Even if you can't actually follow the answers at first, carry on asking and listening until you crack through the painful pattern and realize that hurting yourself with food is not a happy way to live.

Each of us has to walk the path of learning to love ourselves. No one can tell anyone else the 'right' way to do it because our needs are unique. If food is the way you unsuccessfully try to meet your needs and this topic feels too big to tackle now, read the other sections in this book and focus on an aspect of your life—no matter how small—where it's easier for you to be kind and

IF I LOVED MYSELF IN MY FOOD

loving to yourself. Strengthen your self-love in the places where you already meet your needs better and slowly build your confidence to tackle the harder places.

 Pause now, take a breath and say something kind to yourself

Food can be just one of the many places where you practice self-love. In the next section, I share how my children help me practice this.

If I loved myself, how would I choose to use food now?

Wanting a treat

In the car on the way home my children decided to try their luck—as they do—and asked, "Mama, please can we go to the fast-food burger place for a treat?"

They expected me to say no as usual, but I said, "I need to think about it."

They shut up very quickly. I heard one whisper in total amazement to the other, "Don't say *anything*! She's *thinking* about it. She hasn't said *no*!"

The reason I had to think about it was that I also felt like having a food treat—although the thought of putting unidentified processed meat on a chemically preserved white-bread roll with deep-fried reconstituted potatoes and artificially sweetened carbonated liquid chemicals into my body didn't feel great to me. *Maybe I'll let them have a burger and I'll abstain*, I thought. But that was bizarre—I wouldn't choose something for my own body but I'd choose it for the pure, precious bodies of my children? *What kind of a mother am I?* (Let me be *very* clear here: I'm not judging people for allowing their kids to eat fast food. I also do at times. What was strange was being willing to give them something I felt was too unhealthy for *me*.) *What should I do?* I wondered. *We all feel like a food treat, but I don't want to feel uncomfortable afterwards.*

Then I remembered a fast-food place that has fruit smoothies and freshly made food. I told my kids what I'd been thinking and the realization I'd had about my mothering, and they were keen to try the other place—"It's better than nothing," they agreed philosophically.

I felt happy about my decision and we all enjoyed our meal. With his mouth full of his fresh steak wrap and strawberry smoothie, my son said, "Now I know how to get Mama to take us out to eat!"

I felt very nourished by that meal because I'd followed my Truth—and the food was tasty too! But what can you do if a food craving hits hard?

How to love yourself through a craving

When you're craving a particular food and you *know* it's not coming from a place of love but you also know you're going to eat it anyway, acknowledge yourself.

Don't apply willpower—apply love. When we eat this way it's usually to avoid our feelings, so make it safe for yourself to feel. Here's how:

(EXERCISE:) **HOW TO LOVE YOURSELF THROUGH A CRAVING**

Before eating the food you're craving, take five to ten minutes to sit with a pen and paper in a quiet place where you won't be interrupted. Tell yourself, "OK, I see I really want to eat this, and I can. I'll just do this first, and afterwards I can eat without guilt." Then ask yourself these questions and write down the answers:

1. How do I feel right now?
2. What non-food thing would I love to have right now that would genuinely make me feel better? (For example, I'd love to cry, have a nap, have time to myself, feel loved, feel freedom, have something nice for myself, feel safe …)
3. If this food was magic, what would it make me feel?
4. Is there anything I can do for myself right now that will help me feel more like I want to feel?
5. Will eating this food bring me closer or take me further from feeling how I most want to feel?
6. If I loved myself, what would I choose to do now?

After answering these questions honestly and fully (and crying if you need to), if you still want to eat the food, then give yourself *full* permission to do so—and *no* shaming later. Just enjoy it thoroughly.

When your food craving is based on emotion rather than nutrition, what you're actually needing is love and validation. Take the time to check in with yourself. Reflecting on these questions every time you feel the craving for something you wish you didn't will teach you what drives your craving and enable you to give yourself the love and validation you need.

Put these questions on your fridge and make it a fridge full of love.

> **DOWNLOAD** Love yourself through a craving
> www.ifilovedmyself.com/members/chapter-6

A plateful of love

When you serve yourself food, no matter what it is, do so with the care you'd take over the food of a very important person that you love.

If it brings you joy to eat straight from the pot or pan, then do that. But if you normally eat with an attitude that 'it's just me', try this instead: pretend you're serving the food in a restaurant, and take the time and effort to make your plate look appealing. You are serving your most important guest—*you*.

I wish you a tummy full of love.

END OF CHAPTER CHECK IN

- How do you view food now?
- Has how you see food changed in any way through reading this chapter?
- What kind thing would you like to say to yourself about you and food?
- Is there any decision you want to make at this time about listening to your body?

Watch the video again or read the chapter summary to help you clarify your views. Write down your intention for yourself regarding food—perhaps on the chapter summary.

Here's the one-page summary of this chapter to download now to remind yourself of the key points of loving yourself in your food.

DOWNLOAD Chapter 6 summary
www.ifilovedmyself.com/members/chapter-6

Chapter 7

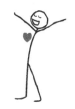

If I loved myself in my Money

Money can buy you a fine dog, but only love can make him wag his tail.
Kinky Friedman

Wealth is the ability to fully experience life.
Henry David Thoreau

SET AN INTENTION FOR THIS CHAPTER NOW

Setting an intention is a powerful way of increasing the effectiveness of what you are doing. Your intention is about your own needs and desired outcomes; it's unique to you and where you are in your life right now. Examples are:
- My intention while reading this chapter is to understand my patterns and choices that don't serve me regarding money and how I can do things differently
- I have the intention to love and value myself with my money
- I intend to learn how to use my money to better meet my needs.

Before you work through the chapter, scan this code to join me for a short video meditation about setting an intention for yourself and your money.

You can also access the meditation through this link:
www.ifilovedmyself.com/members/chapter-7

What's a chapter on money doing in a book like this?

Money is a self-love thing. I don't mean that people who have little money have poor self-worth and those with a lot of money feel good about themselves—we've all heard stories of very unhappy wealthy people. In fact, tabloids thrive on that, probably because many of us need proof that we're not less worthy than those who seem 'successful.' Having or not having money is neither here nor there. It's the *relationship* we have with our money—the way we feel about it and how we use it (or let it use us)—that reflects how we value ourselves, set our boundaries and open ourselves to giving and receiving in the world. Money says a lot about our love for ourselves and how we feel about our worth.

Money is complicated—our life experiences, childhood, family history, culture and socio-economic circumstances all feed directly into our relationship with money. We have stories about money: those with money have power; those without money are vulnerable; those who don't care about money are anarchists; those who want more money are greedy … The stories we buy into dictate how we dance with this life energy we call Money.

In this chapter you'll meet people who looked at their relationship with money, saw how it reflected their relationship with themselves and then made choices from greater self-love. Ask yourself, *How do I see money?*

Does your relationship with money reflect something about how you value yourself?

If you loved yourself, how would you choose to view your money?

Money and food

The way we deal with our money is often similar to how we deal with our food.

Gina has been dealing with food issues for many years. She always feels stressed that there won't be enough, and this is partly because she grew up with many siblings, who grabbed all the food as soon as it was put on the table. She was the quiet, shy one and was often left without as much as the others. She didn't go hungry, but the fear of not getting food was deeply entrenched.

Another part of her food dance is that she tends to disconnect from her emotions. She's started to realize that each time she turns away from her Truth, she offers herself compensation for losing something so important. So she has the glass of wine or the cream cake or the chocolate—as though she is important to herself after all. The problem is that her good feeling doesn't last long because it's a replacement for her real need. Then, in another unhelpful attempt to meet her needs, she punishes her body with all sorts of crazy diets.

This chapter is about money, so why am I telling you about Gina's food habits? Because when it comes to money, she does the very same thing. She lends money to her friends, who seldom pay her back, and are then too uncomfortable to spend time with her. Gina supports her sister, who finds it difficult to keep a job, and so Gina has less money to spend on herself. She regularly buys clothes and school equipment for the children of the woman who cleans her house, but this woman often has dramas at home that mean she leaves work early or doesn't come in at all.

Gina gives and gives and gives—and gets little in return. She feels hurt and unimportant to the people she helps, but pushes aside her feelings and chooses to give yet more. In this way, she turns away from her Truth and leaves herself 'hungry' because she doesn't attend to her own needs. Desperate for something to make her feel better, she then spends large amounts of money, which makes her feel better for a while. But then she starts to feel guilty and stressed about not having enough money, and the cycle begins again.

Anyone reading this would say Gina should stop giving away her money but she does it because she's trying to meet her needs for love, approval and attention. Her child-self is deeply wishing that everyone would stop grabbing her 'food' and would care enough to see her and ask what she wants. But Gina is actually the one taking advantage of her own giving nature—other people's love and attention is always auxiliary to our own. To meet her real need to be noticed and to matter, Gina must notice herself and ask herself what she needs.

Are your food and money habits similar in any way?

If I loved myself, how would I choose to use my money now?

Get real

Brent comes to see me one day in a state of distress. His movements are jerky, he's breathing fast and isn't able to maintain eye contact. He's spent money he doesn't have on something he doesn't need, and now he has even more debt.
"Why did I do it?" he says in a low moan, gazing at the floor.
We spend five minutes taking slow, deliberate, deep stomach breaths—this soothes the autonomic nervous system by sending the message there's no real danger. Then we gently explore what triggered his spending.

He'd been with friends who earn much more than he does, and he'd felt inadequate and small—a familiar trigger for him. After dinner he'd gone home and seen an email promotion for the car he'd been lusting after. In that brief shining moment, he'd felt everything would be better if he just had that car. So he'd signed on the dotted line and messaged everyone about it. Now, in the cold light of day, he feels completely sick with fear—he can't afford the payments. We speak it through for a while and then I ask him the Love question.

His response is, "If I loved myself, I wouldn't have spent the money."

While that may be true, there are two problems with this answer. The first is that he looks completely woebegone when he says it, and that is *not* how our Truth feels. His expression is the result of self-judgment in this moment. The second is that he's using wishful thinking—which has its place, but not when you're trying to get out of a pickle.

I tell him: "If you hadn't spent the money, you'd have done something else reckless because you were trying to avoid your painful feelings in that moment. The real question to ask yourself is, 'Now that I've taken an action that brings me difficulty, if I loved myself, what would I do now?'"

He nods. "How do I love myself even after I've done something so stupid?"

I smile. His humor is a good sign that he's calming down.

Then he continues: "I guess I'd say to myself, 'I'm learning. This isn't great, but it'll probably help me realize that money won't fix my self-esteem issues. I won't do something like this again—it's a really awful feeling. If I loved myself, I would pat myself on the head kindly, keep saying reassuring things and start looking for a way to get out of the mess I made while I felt scared."

Brent connected money with success and worth. The next section has a few questions to help you explore whether you do this too.

Does money define success?

Money is commonly linked with our definition of success or failure; people are even described as successes or failures based on their wealth. Apparently, this emerged from how financial institutions rated people for investment risks: they introduced into our vocabulary concepts such as, "He's a zero/he'll amount to nothing/he's a failure/he's a bad bet". Prior to this, the idea of a person being 'a failure' was not in our collective consciousness. A person's business venture or attempt could fail, but the *person* was not a failure.

EXERCISE: WHAT ARE YOUR RATING SCALES?

1. How much of a role does money play in your definition of success and why?
2. What happens to love when you define a person's worth by how much money they have?
3. Do you think every person who has made a lot of money fulfills your personal criteria for being a 'successful person'?
4. Do you know anyone with little money who you think of as being a 'successful person' anyway?

If I loved myself, how would I define success for myself?

 Pause now, take a breath and say something kind to yourself

Money highlights what's already there

There are many different money dynamics, and ways in which money reflects our feelings of self-worth. Perhaps you can identify your own patterns after reading the stories below.

Kareem doesn't believe in himself. He doubts everything he does and occasionally says that he hates himself. He never has 'enough' money to feel secure in the world—it's hard to feel secure when your own self is out to get you!

Shana doesn't like herself either, but she has lots of money. She uses her money to apologize for her existence on this planet. She gives to charity and is over-generous to people. Despite this, she doesn't have many real friends because her insecurity is difficult to be around. This validates her belief that she's boring and that people don't like her. To try to make it better, she hosts lavish events but is left feeling just as lonely. Her money keeps her from having to face her vulnerability—any time she sees people's discomfort with her, she 'throws money at the problem'. It's hard to be liked when you don't like yourself.

Jason also has a lot of money, but he has many good friends and colleagues. A vibrant man, he's often the life of the party. He likes himself well enough, but he tends to ignore his Truth if it means he'll let someone else down. He'd rather let himself down—that doesn't feel as serious to him. His money protects him from having to be very strict about his boundaries because if he gives too much he doesn't really feel it financially. However, as other people follow his example and let him down rather than themselves, he's starting to feel used and to question if people like him or just his money. Asking himself that is beginning to cause radical changes in his relationships—both with himself and with others.

Love yourself with your money

The role of money in your life can be to enhance and affirm the genuine love and appreciation you feel for your own sweet Self and how you express in the world. Here are two very important questions to ask yourself:

- Do I use my money to love myself, or to punish and restrict myself?
- Do I use my money to affirm my worth, or to judge myself for not being good enough?

The way to tell which one you more commonly lean towards is to answer this:

- When I think of my money, do I get feelings of openness, potential and joy, or do I get sinking feelings of self-judgment, limitation and hopelessness?
- Do my feelings when I think of money become lighter and wider, or do they weight me down and tighten me?

Jared, in the next story, has very strong beliefs about his money and his worth—with awful consequences.

If you loved yourself, what would you choose to do or say about your money that would feel lighter to you?

> **CHECK IN**
>
> How do you feel about you and money right now compared with at the start of this chapter? Has anything changed in how you view your money? Say something kind to yourself right now. Then keep reading. Try to do this a few times throughout this chapter. By the end you and your money may have become closer friends.

Will money give me worth?

Jared desperately wants money. He believes his lack of money affirms his poor opinion of himself, and imagines money will meet his need to feel powerful in the world. He gambles compulsively, hoping to win big and make all his problems go away. He borrows money from everyone who's willing, gets into trouble with loan sharks and isn't able to pay his rent. His girlfriend of many years is constantly financially stressed – which makes him feel even less 'like a man'. He tries one impulsive business scheme after another, but none hit the jackpot. He owes so much money. He finds himself lying, stealing and cheating just to keep ahead of the debt that's chasing him. One day in desperation he pawns his car and takes the cash to the casino.

Life has an interesting way of answering our calls for help. It gives us what we need—and because we have free will, what we do with what we receive is up to us.

Jared wins a lot of money that day in the casino. He wins enough to buy back his car and pay off his debt. However, instead of cashing in his chips, over the course of a few more hours he gambles it all away. The truth is that Jared can't allow himself to have so much money. He doesn't feel he's worth it.

I find Jared's story painful—even more so because what Jared really needs is just to know he has worth, and to feel loved and accepted. He could have that at any time—it was never about the money.

At some point, most of us will deny ourselves the very thing we most want, even when it's there for the taking. We seek intimacy, but create an argument when we have time alone with our loved one. We want to eat well, and then get too busy to choose healthy food options. We want to do creative projects, but play on our phone when we have spare time …

If you notice yourself repeatedly seeking something you feel you can't get, ask yourself, *What is my real need? What do I believe I'll feel if I have that thing?* Your answer will show what you really need. Then do something that will bring you the *feelings* you seek.

If I loved myself, what would I choose to allow myself now?

Choosing a story of enough

Money concerns are not necessarily related to whether there's enough money to survive—even very rich people sometimes live with the fear of not having enough. Concern around money simply means there's a stressful story attached to having enough money. I grew up in a family with fear stories about money, only some of which were based on our real survival needs. I also had friends in whose homes money was not a concern. I saw their attitudes and preferred their relaxed assumption that there'd always be enough. I wanted that for myself.

Looking back now, I see that throughout my life I've made choices to ensure that money isn't something I worry about. That doesn't mean I've made choices that would bring me the most money—I remember one of my university lecturers mumbling, "We don't become psychologists to get rich." But I've made choices that meant money wouldn't cause worry for me. On my own initiative I got myself a job when I was fifteen, because I liked the independence of having my own money and not adding to my family's money concerns. It made me feel more relaxed about money. It made money joyful for me. In my twenties I suddenly got a job that earned much more money than I was used to, and I took the opportunity to buy things I needed and spent money I wouldn't have before. Then that job unexpectedly ended, I was left with very little money again and no savings. I didn't like that, so I decided to use my money differently the next time I had a lot of it flowing in. That decision also made me feel more relaxed about money. Nowadays when I reflect on my relaxed money stories I want to giggle with glee—this is what I so longed for as a child. It has little to do with how much money I have, and a lot to do with how I *feel* about what I have.

In my practice and my life now I'm pretty relaxed about money and I'm so grateful that it's something with which I'm increasingly comfortable. I know I'll always have enough—and if I don't, I'll make a plan. Through trial and error, I've learned I can trust myself to make sure I have enough of what I need. My trust in myself means I trust my money. I feel very loved by myself in this regard.

Clients who engage with me sometimes feel stressed about my relaxed attitude—which offers a great opportunity to explore their stories about money. I specifically remember one person looking at me with great concern for my professionalism. In our first session he asked exactly how and when he needed to pay, and my response was that he could do so in the way that best suited him. From his expression of distaste it was clear he wasn't planning on coming back to this crackpot! I told him I'd send an invoice at month's end and trust him to pay weekly or monthly.
"But how do you know I'll pay?" he demanded.
"This is a relationship," I replied. "There's connection and there needs to be trust. People pay me. It's part of our relationship."

He and I have had a beautiful journey since then. He's always paid me, and does so the way that suits him best. We've since laughed about his distrust of me in that first session—and the fear my trust raised in him.

Money is not a dirty word.

It's a symbol of life energy and how we use it in the world. It shows us how much we allow ourselves to exist and be acknowledged. It's a real indicator of what we use our energy for and who we think deserves what. It's a relationship that'll go through ups and downs—both are opportunities to learn how to love yourself more. Whether you have a lot or a little, too much or not enough, money helps you see your self-love choices.

If you loved yourself, how would it affect your trust with your money? What story would you choose for yourself?

Would you do anything for money?

One of the strangest things about money in our society is that we've somehow made it more powerful than anything else in our world. So many things in our culture are skewed because of it. Some religions teach that poverty equals piousness, yet religious leaders and institutions can be corrupted by money; presidents are elected because they can pay for expensive campaigns; children are accepted to schools because their families can donate more; cutting-edge medical advances are only offered to those who can pay the price; wise elders who no longer earn money are pushed aside; teachers and public healthcare workers (the people in charge of our collective health and well-being) are paid minimum wages ... We're pretty much a societal mess when it comes to money.

The weirdest part of the power our society gives money is its ability to override other truths. Someone can be 'bought off'. What does that mean? It refers to someone turning away from their Truth, self-love and integrity in order to gain money. Somehow we accept the idea that getting money is a good enough reason to not listen to your own Truth. So money can be a direct catalyst for someone behaving in a non-self-loving way. In some way or another most of us do this in our daily lives. We might buy battery-chicken eggs because they're cheaper, or cheap plastic stuff even though it contributes to environmental degradation. We might accept the stressful brief, or put up with the abusive boss rather than lose money.

We've been taught that money is extremely important, but it's actually just a tool to love yourself well.

If you see it as a material expression of your energy, you can earn it by doing things that feel good to you and lovingly use it to make sure you have all you need to thrive. So ask yourself now:

- How do I see money?
- How much money would it take for me to not listen to myself?
- Where do I already compromise my Truth because of money?
- What's the real cost to me?

Money is *never* a good enough reason to turn away from your Truth, self-love and integrity. The cost is always higher than the benefits.

If I loved myself, how would I choose to love money differently now?

 Pause now, take a breath and say something kind to yourself

I feel like an imposter

Tara grew up in a well-off family. Then her family lost all their money and she experienced a painful and humiliating stretch of poverty that badly impacted her family relationships and left deep scars on her feelings of self-worth. Now she has a high-earning job and the money stresses her out—she wants to enjoy it, but the fear of losing it lurks constantly. She finds it difficult to relax into having money. Like so many others who've gained wealth or status, she feels she's pretending to be rich and if people could see the real her, it would be the poor, humiliated girl she once was. She's hired people to help her look after her money because it makes her so anxious to engage with it herself.

As she heals and her self-worth increases, her relationship with money is beginning to change. She's starting to feel proud of her worth and capacity. She's striving to learn that she'll be fine no matter what—whether she keeps her wealth or loses it all. She's learning to love herself and act accordingly.

Here are two questions Tara's story inspired me to add:

If I loved myself, how much money would I allow myself to fearlessly earn?

If I loved myself, how would I allow myself to genuinely enjoy the money I have?

Can she buy love?

Suki and her sister are complete opposites when it comes to their relationship with money. When they received pocket money as children, Suki's sister had an amazing knack for stretching it out over a long time. Suki, on the other hand, would immediately go to the corner shop and spend the whole lot, gorging on sweets and happily sharing them with friends and family for the rest of the day. Then she'd be left with no money and no sweets for the rest of the week. She always felt there wasn't enough—except for those brief, wonderful periods where she had lots.

As an adult, Suki has noticed that she gets rid of her money as soon as it comes in. While enjoying the moment is a wonderful part of who she is, she's realized it's anxiety that makes her spend all her money. In therapy we agree she'll practice having savings and keeping unspent money in her wallet to notice what feelings emerge.

Slowly she unpacks this psychological suitcase and sees how as a young child she felt less than her sister, who was clever and popular (and always had money!). Suki sees how she tried to buy her sister's love and attention by sharing, and how hurt she felt when her sister didn't share with her, saying, "You've spent all yours. This is mine." Young Suki felt her sister didn't care about her, which chipped away at her feeling of worth.

Now, years later, as Suki practices new money behavior, these anxieties and doubts have emerged from where they've been hiding. When she sees this, she decides to love her younger Self and meet her real needs. Step by step, she practices making her spending choices from a place of self-love, and now she's even chosen to have a savings account! It's a journey, but Suki no longer hides her true needs for love and connection behind money.

If I loved myself, what would I choose to spend my money on?

How we quietly repeat our patterns

Zorell's family has a long history of not having enough money. Everyone has had to work very hard because of bad money decisions, and he remembers his parents being stressed and overworked for most of his childhood. They seemed absent to him, but now he can see they were worried about money all the time. Part of him feels money has robbed him of his parents.

He has an angry yet longing relationship with money. He stores it up so he won't be like his family, but he does it in a way that deprives him of the comforts that money can bring. One day he realizes, "I think I'm saving too much! I put so much into my savings that I'm always worried about not having enough for my daily needs. Then I tell myself I can't have stuff because it's too expensive. But I *do* have the money for it. Why don't I let myself enjoy it?"

It's amazing how we repeat the patterns we learned when we were small. In his intense effort to make sure he isn't stressed about money, Zorell finds himself stressed about money. He's recreated the pattern where lack of money means he isn't loved and cared for in the way he needs. He's an 'absent caregiver' to himself.

His self-love answers? "If I loved myself, I'd save a little less. I'd use my money to show myself I'm listening to and caring for me."

If you loved yourself, what money pattern would you change now?

Stories we tell ourselves about rich people

"Money corrupts people," Mikhail says to me one day. He's been very successful in business, but never quite reaches what he perceives to be the upper echelons of earning. "There are points where you have to sell your soul to make the really big money. I'm not prepared to do that."

"I don't like rich people," Sandra says when we explore why she doesn't ever earn as much as she'd like. "They're cold, uncaring snobs. I don't ever want to be like that."

If you loved yourself, what stories would you tell yourself about rich people?

Why she can't have money

Anushka grew up in a low-income area with crime and abuse all around. She's tried very hard to earn enough to move away, but can't yet afford it. Everyone around her is poor and struggling.

Her family coped in their everyday life—but no one was doing well financially, and it was regular practice for people to borrow money to make it to the end of the month. As a teenager, Anushka noticed that people with lighter skin at her school tended to have more money. So she developed a story within herself that people with darker skins usually have less money, and everything she saw in society confirmed this. Without realizing it, she settled into a story that she'd never be wealthy because of her dark skin. Anushka can see that she's now living out this story.

"If you loved yourself, how would you choose to view money?" I ask her.
She thinks for a long time, and I can see inner battles waging within her. "I think, if I loved myself more ... I'd see myself the same way I see white people. That I could also have easy access to money and live well in a nice house somewhere safe." Then she pauses and feels that out. "I think I'll need some time to get used to that idea," she says—but she's smiling.

If you loved yourself, how would you choose to see money and you now?

A story about procrastination

At the end of each month, I sit down to do my accounts. Basically, I check what money is owed, what's come in, who's paid and needs an invoice, who still needs to pay and what invoices need to be sent out for the month just ended. Luckily, resistance to admin is on my list of 'Problems I don't have'. (That's a very useful and reassuring list to have. I learned about it from my mother. We spend so much of our time focusing on our problems that we sometimes feel we have *all* the problems there are to have. When you hear of a particular problem you *don't* experience, take mental note and enjoy your wonderful self for *not* having that problem. It puts your problems into some kind of perspective. Give the things you *don't* struggle with some loving appreciation.)

So this is a problem I don't have but nevertheless, a while back I found myself procrastinating when it was accounts time. It wasn't obvious resistance at first—there were just a lot of other things to attend to and accounts moved lower down the list. After a while though, I noticed that I was regularly putting other things first and becoming adolescent about it: *Oh*, man. *There's this thing I HAVE to do and I want to do those OTHER things but I can't because of THIS thing!* Cue dramatic eye roll.

There are things in my life I do The Eye-Roll about, but as admin isn't usually one of them, I realized something was up. There were clearly some needs not being met, so it was time to ask the Love question. My head, of course, knew I 'should' do my accounts, but something was interfering and I wanted to hear what my heart had to say about it. So I sat and felt it out. I meditated, listened to the feelings in my body and asked myself what they were trying to tell me. I could sense myself feeling angry and disempowered that I 'had' to do something instead of being free to choose. I could see I had a need to feel free from obligations but that still didn't make things clear. What had changed?

I asked, "If I loved myself, what would I choose to do now?"

Perhaps I thought my answer would give me permission to slack off—but as I keep saying, when it comes to listening to your Truth, expect the unexpected. What came quietly to my mind and heart was, "If I loved myself, I'd send out invoices for my services because it's an acknowledgement of my worth." The answer came with that chest-opening, spontaneous relaxation and elevated happy feeling that signifies my Truth. It also made my eyes tear up. But it was such a surprising answer because my head had already been trying to get me to do that, so why had I been resisting? What was all the fuss about?

Slowly it became clear to me that putting off my accounts had made me feel more and more unacknowledged, and even somewhat insecure about my worth. It's very affirming to say, "I value what I do, and this is what I charge for it." When I wasn't happily saying it about myself, a part of me started to rebel! So, like a child who refuses to eat because she's so overwhelmed with hunger, I'd refused to do the very thing I most wanted and needed.

I've taken that information I received from myself and put it to self-loving use. Now as each month end rolls around I get a bit excited about spending a couple of hours affirming myself. When I feel resentful or resistant—which sometimes still happens—I remind my inner rebel of the loved feeling I get when I affirm myself. She just wants to know she's loved. The accounts still get sent out as they always have been, but the experience has gone from something just to get done to something loving, joyous and affirming. There's no difference on the outside but what a huge, massive, wonderful difference for me on the inside!

Shifting your perspective can be the key that changes how you experience a situation. Sandile, in the next story, faced a sharp challenge in this regard.

Guilt for having too much

Sandile has just got a raise at work. You'd think that would be a good thing, but it's brought up some real stress for him.

"I feel so uncomfortable having so much money," he tells me. "Part of me is really happy and excited, but another part wants to apologize to everyone."

Of course I ask why he'd need to, and out comes his story.

"I grew up very poor. We lived in a two-room shack—my mother, five children, my father and my uncle. My mom worked as a cleaner and she did her best, but there was never enough. My father couldn't find regular work and my uncle just drank and caused trouble. We didn't have enough money for school or clothes or food. We were always getting notes from the school asking us to pay something towards fees, but we just didn't have it.

"I'm the second-eldest boy. My oldest sister had to stay home from the age of twelve to help with the younger children. My oldest brother left school at fifteen to work in construction so we could have more money coming in. I did well, so the family put aside money to keep me in school. Later I got a scholarship to a better school in the suburbs. I needed money to get there and back—it was an hour away—and for uniform and books. It all cost so much. The scholarship covered most of it but there were always extra things we were supposed to do—like bring a cake for a bake sale and stuff like that. I always felt bad asking for anything extra.

"But I was so happy getting out of the settlement every day and meeting rich people and learning new things. I did well but I had to pretend to fit in. I worked very hard. I couldn't let my family down after all they were doing to keep me there. Then I graduated and got a bursary for university. I'm the first in our family to finish high school—going to university had been an unreachable dream. I did well and got a job and now most of my salary goes to my family. I've bought them a house and a car, and I make sure they have what they need. But I got all these opportunities while my two older siblings worked to help us survive. They didn't get an education. And my two younger siblings couldn't try for a better school because all the spare money was going to *my* school needs. I got all this good stuff and they suffered.

"Now I have an apartment of my own and a nice car and a good job, and I eat nice food, and I feel guilty, guilty, *guilty*. With this promotion I get even *more* money and I want to throw up from the stress. Why did I get all the nice stuff? How do I enjoy it when they don't have what I have? Nothing can make up for not having an education. They lost out on that—it's something I can never repay. I know I'm their pension plan, but that feels like a prison sentence. How many will I have to support? My parents and uncle and brothers and sisters and their children and theirs? I don't own my life. I'm like a cash machine. I wish I could take this money and give it all to them and be free. But I can't because I can never repay this debt of what I got and they didn't."

At this point Sandile's voice breaks and he can no longer hold it in. He puts his face in his hands and sobs, his thin shoulders hunched up and shaking. He looks so forlorn, I have to hold back my urge to gather him in my arms and rock him like a baby. When his release eases, we talk more about his concerns, and when it's appropriate I introduce the idea of loving yourself—in particular, that money shows us how we love ourselves. He finds this fascinating and asks a lot of questions. His whole demeanor shifts, as if someone's switched on a light in his face.

"So I could use money to love myself rather than punish myself ..." he says thoughtfully at one point. At the end of our session he thanks me profusely and earnestly.

I didn't get to see Sandile again, so I don't know what happened with him or what choices he made. His initial despair and then his shining, hopeful face at the end of our session touched me deeply. As a therapist I know that ideally Sandile needs to find a way to come to terms with what happened to him and to his loved ones and that's not easy. It was unfair and the effects are still ongoing. His relationships with his family and community will always be affected in some way by their differences in education levels, life experiences and wealth. It's a loss of identity and community and something he has to learn to manage.

It's a very difficult journey to step out of poverty while your loved ones remain in it and it becomes a thousand-fold more complicated when they sacrificed to help you do it. It makes it difficult to believe you have the right to love yourself. I hope Sandile will one day realize that he wasn't to blame for the family's hardships. The socioeconomic situation meant they probably would have struggled even if he hadn't gone to those schools. He, and so many like him, has a version of survivor's guilt. The way he might find peace is to remember that he was as much at the mercy of the situation as they were. It's easy to compare lifestyles and decide one is easier than the other but both sides of this situation are hard. Sandile acknowledges his family's hardships but he also needs to acknowledge his own. Money and material comfort don't take away pain. Love does.

At the end of the day, whatever our circumstances are, we are each responsible for how we choose to live, react and behave. Sandile's task is to accept that how he chooses to manage his community's needs and expectations is up to him—and how they choose to manage the situation from their side is their responsibility. It will serve everyone if Sandile can make choices that are loving of himself as well as of them.

I tried to imagine what self-love would look like in his circumstances, and this is the fantasy follow-up I created: When he comes back to see me, Sandile is a different man. Smiling broadly, this extraordinary man tells me that he'd gone home, figured out his budget with his salary increase and then approached his family members individually. He explained to each of them the concept that money is a way to love yourself, and asked what their dream was. Then he began to put a plan in place to support each of them in taking the actions they need to achieve their particular dream. "This is how I want to use my money and my education," he says, sitting back like a man in his power. "And now I want to earn as much as I can because I can help my family's dreams come true. This is what I'll do with my money. This is how I'll love myself. I feel free for the first time since this whole thing began— now I'm glad I got those opportunities. I was just the one going ahead to give the others a hand. All our dreams can come true—it's not too late for any of us."

Imagine a world in which we understood money as a tool to love ourselves genuinely and follow our Truth? Imagine a world in which we all help each other fulfill our dreams.

If you loved yourself, what would you choose to say to yourself about what you have now?

How much money do you need?

Yona had a job, a house and a relationship until things happened and she found herself without any of those. She lived where she could, had to ask for financial support from friends and family, and constantly found herself staring at an empty wallet wondering how she was going to make it through the day, never mind the week. What amazed her was that each time she found herself at her wit's end, something surprising and wonderful came along to tend to her needs. Sometimes it was selling something she'd made, sometimes an offer of a place to stay, and other times money that would suddenly come her way.

Yona tells me that she's begun to question how much we really need to get by. How much money do we need to feel safe and supported in the world? She's interested in the traveling teachers in India, who're completely taken care of by whichever community is hosting them at the time.

"Perhaps you can love yourself even without money ..." I venture.

She gazes at me. "I'm learning so much about money through all this, but I can't quite see the connection between money and loving myself."

"To me it's the same thing," I say. "You've been learning more about yourself and more about money. You've been listening to yourself and to money. You've been learning to accept and love yourself more and allow yourself to engage with money in a more open and allowing way. It's the same process. It's about loving yourself."

She looks at me. "I feel like my whole body is blinking," she says. "Like little eyes all over my body are blinking at this new idea."

Your spending choices reveal what you believe in

Money, like food, is something we flow into our system. If your money is part of your energy system, whatever you choose to spend your money on becomes part of your energetic body. So it makes sense to ask yourself, *If I loved myself, would I choose to include this in my system?*

What you spend your money on shows what you believe in and support.

To believe and support something means you want to strengthen it in the world and include it in your daily life and Self. Think about what you spend your money on: big things like cars and homes, and smaller things like food and clothes and treats. Are they things you want to strengthen in your body and in the world? Do you believe in and support the things you spend your money on? Do they enhance or diminish your self-love? If you want to clarify which it is for you, ask, *Does this make me feel loved?*

EXERCISE: THOUGHT-PROVOKING QUESTIONS TO ASK ABOUT YOUR SPENDING

- Is there anything you spend money on and feel guilty about after? Why? If you loved yourself, what would you choose to do differently?
- Is there anything you spend your money on and feel joyful about? Do you do it enough? If you loved yourself, how often would you do this?
- What's a treat for you? Why does it feel like a treat? Do you need to use money to feel this way? If you loved yourself, what would you do to increase this good feeling?
- Is there anything you buy only because it's cheap or you can afford it—but if

you could afford more, you wouldn't flow more of your money there? If you loved yourself, would you change anything?
- How do you feel about other people's money—when they have a lot, or when they have a little? What beliefs come up when you think of how other people manage their money? Think of spendthrifts you know, and then think of misers—what judgment and fears emerge?
- How do you feel about beggars? What do beggars make you aware of about your money stories? Ask yourself, *If I loved myself what story would I tell myself when I'm faced with someone begging for money?*
- Do you know anyone you consider money-healthy?
- How much fear do you have attached to money? Fear is a love-blocker. (See "In Your Self" for more on this.) So if you had no fear about money, how might you feel about it?
- If your money was connected to self-love, how might it change your attitude and story about money?

If I loved myself in my money, what would I choose to do now?

Deprivation is not about money

A person can have endless money and feel deprived, or none at all and feel rich. That's because money is just a symbol, a tool—it can't meet our real needs.

The feeling of wealth, of having enough, actually connects to being present in any moment. You meet your needs when you give full and loving attention and appreciation to what you already have right now—and then you feel rich.

The most effective way to counteract the feeling of deprivation is to practice appreciation. What's in your bank account has nothing to do with that.

If I loved myself, how would I create the feeling of wealth for myself in this moment?

END OF CHAPTER CHECK IN

- What are your views on money now?
- Have they changed in any way through reading this chapter?
- What would you like to say to yourself about you and money?
- Is there any decision you'd like to make at this time about your money?

Watch the video again and read the chapter summary to help you clarify your views. Write down your intention for yourself and money from now on—perhaps on the chapter summary.

Here's the one-page summary of this chapter to download now to remind yourself of the key points of loving yourself in your money.

DOWNLOAD Chapter 7 summary
www.ifilovedmyself.com/members/chapter-7

Chapter 8

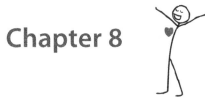

If I loved myself in my Sex

There is a supernal intelligence behind sexual arousal, the true purpose of which is to create for us ecstatic experiences of our own divinity.
John Maxwell Taylor

To experience the most profound levels of sexual ecstasy, we must be willing to release, even if only temporarily, the drive for explosive orgasms and surrender to a quest for self-discovery and healing.
Michael Mirdad

> **SET AN INTENTION FOR THIS CHAPTER NOW**
>
> Setting an intention is a powerful way of increasing the effectiveness of what you are doing. Your intention is about your own needs and desired outcomes; it's unique to you and where you are in your life right now. Examples might be:
> - My intention while reading this chapter is to see my patterns and choices that don't serve me regarding sex and how I might do things differently
> - I have the intention to love and value myself in sex
> - I intend to learn how to listen to and honor my own needs better during sex.
>
>  Before you work through the chapter, scan this code to join me for a short video meditation about setting an intention for yourself and your sex.
>
> You can also access the meditation through this link:
> **www.ifilovedmyself.com/members/chapter-8**

Truth in love 'n sex

Sex is a place where practicing self-loving choices is both brave and tricky. The Truth that emerges might not always be welcome, and we're so used to overriding it that learning to be connected to ourselves while engaging physically with another can be a real challenge. How often during sex—with yourself or your partner—do you focus more on the fantasy in your mind than the sensations in your own body—how it feels, what you like, what you don't ...

We're very exposed when we engage sexually with another person. It's vulnerable. That's probably why, for many people, sex raises anxiety. In the chapter on relationships in "In Your Self", I explain that intimacy is a space in which you're seen by another and because of that you see yourself more clearly. During sex—besides the fact that you mostly don't wear clothes—you have the chance to not wear any roles, disguises or masks. These have their place in the sexual arena, but when it comes to real, intimate sex, it's just you there. Anything that veils your Truth from yourself or your partner hinders the transformative, heart-opening experience that sex with a connected partner can be.

The quality of the sex you have depends greatly on the quality of your connection to yourself and to your partner.

People who fear intimacy might find connected sex to be threatening. They may prefer sex to be a physical act for fun and release; afterwards, there's no deep closeness or expansion of Self—definitely no cuddling. A good workout at the gym could feel almost as good—and less messy. On the other hand, people who crave intimacy find disconnected sex unsatisfying. In fact, to be distant from yourself and the other in an act that's all about closeness can feel emotionally painful.

Masturbation is potentially also a spiritual and sensory journey of self-discovery.

During masturbation, you get to know yourself better, and feel more connected to and loving of yourself, your body and the world in general. It can be a physical experience of real self-love. It's a pity we're not taught this. In fact, many people aren't even present to themselves while they masturbate—they're looking at porn or thinking of something external that arouses them rather than being aroused by their own body. The disconnected terms we use to describe masturbating are so telling: for example, 'getting off'. Getting off what? Imagine if instead you heard someone say, "Oh, that guy's always going within."

In this chapter the focus is on connected sex. Self-love, listening to your needs and following your Truth are fundamental requirements for satisfying connected sex.

So let's get into the bedroom and explore this terrain of making self-loving choices during sexual intimacy. As this is just one chapter in our book, we don't have plenty of time for foreplay. But I'll make a few suggestive remarks and flirt with certain concepts—hopefully enough to get your juices flowing for loving yourself during sex.

Taking off your clothes

Taking off your clothes in front of someone is such an exposing moment—it's literal intimacy.

Sometimes we're so hung up about our bodies that it becomes difficult to relax and be present enough to listen to our real needs during sex.

If you're obsessing about your cellulite, weird nipples, penis size, rough skin, hairiness, flabby tummy, pimples on your bum, saggy breasts ... you can't let yourself enjoy the moment. You're not loving every part of you. Sex is all about the body—and not at all about the body. The main players during sex are actually sensation, emotion, energy and thought. The body is the vehicle for the connection, but it cannot take the place of the connection.

Have you ever felt embarrassed for not looking like the Photo-shopped images in magazines? Those images are so powerful: even though you may *know* they're fake, you still find yourself comparing your body to them. Even celebrities say at times they don't recognize themselves in those photographs. Look around the changing rooms at the gym or go to a nudist resort—you'll be reassured by the many shapes and sizes.

Your body is just fine as it is.

When you don't accept your own body as it is, it's difficult to imagine someone else could. So women keep on their bra or nightie during sex, men put their pants on right afterwards, some people will only have sex in the dark or lie in a certain more flattering position, others won't walk to the toilet naked so their partner doesn't see their bum … The methods of hiding what we deem to be shameful are countless. We all want to be loved as we are—stretch marks, warts and all. For that, we need to begin with accepting ourselves and not judging those things as 'bad'. You're blessed to have a body, and in real life none of our bodies are Photo-shopped.

If you lived in a totally safe and accepting world that didn't dictate how a body 'should' look, what would you feel about your body?

Think about a part of your body you feel uncomfortable or ashamed about, and ask yourself, "If I loved myself, what would I choose to say to myself about this part of my body?"

What is the most empowered way you can imagine getting naked in front of a stranger?

If I loved myself, what would I choose to say to myself about my body?

 Pause now, take a breath and say something kind to yourself

The penis and vagina have intelligence

Sex and sensuality are opportunities to feast on our senses and celebrate ourselves. Our whole body is a sensory organ. Each part of our body is particularly good at some type of sensing. Our skin receives touch; our chest area perceives emotion; our breasts, penis, vagina, womb, testicles, brain, nose, eyes, tongue and ears all tune into their own area of sensory interest.

In Chapter 5 on body and health, I spoke about how each part of your body stores and represents aspects of yourself. I gave a few exercises to help you learn to listen to what is represented by your body (see page 129). In the arena of sex and sensuality, I recommend that you practice listening to your body parts as you engage with them for the sake of pleasure and connection.

In the practice of sacred sexuality known as Tantra, it's acknowledged that a penis, a vagina, breasts, etc., all have their own kind of intelligence. They're not just tools to use (or abuse). What does this mean?

A penis or vagina is a wise and wonderful aspect of yourself with which to engage.

IF YOU LOVED YOURSELF, WHAT WOULD YOU DO NOW?

In Tantra workshops, men and women are asked to have conversations with their penis or vagina. While this makes most people nervous at first, these conversations often bring deep healing and connection with Self. Try the next exercise to experience it for yourself.

EXERCISE: A CONVERSATION WITH YOUR PENIS OR VAGINA

1. Sit quietly, fully clothed or naked, in a place where you won't be interrupted. Take three slow, deep breaths. On your third deep breath, hold it at the top of the inhale for as long as you can before releasing.
2. Gently bring your mental attention to your penis or vagina. Just allow yourself to sit in stillness while you hold this awareness. Notice what thoughts and feelings come up, but don't engage with them much. Simply observe your own reactions.
3. Make an intention to communicate with your penis or vagina (like turning towards a person with the intention to speak to them). Notice how it responds to your intention, as you would assess someone when you approach to talk to them. Is there a sense of willingness and delight in communicating with you? A wariness? A feeling of anger and resentment? Fear and reluctance? This indicates the condition of the love relationship between your penis or vagina and You.
4. Begin talking. Say hello. Sense the response. Ask why it feels the way it does towards you. Ask how it feels about you talking to it now. Ask if there's something it would like to tell you. Ask any questions you may have. Tell it what you feel you want to say. Engage with it as an intelligent, dear friend who's on your team. See what emerges.

When you make love—with yourself or with another—be aware that it is a deep and multidimensional communication between yourself and all your sensory receptors as well as with your partner and all of theirs. Sex is often portrayed as disconnected body parts chafing together for physical release. We miss out on so much when we disconnect from our skin, breasts, penis or vagina in this way.

Sex is designed to be a communing with Self—a chance to open to experience the magnificent orchestra of your whole body and being.

If you're not sure how to do this, keep communicating with your body parts, ask the Love question and follow the guidance you receive.

Nyall, in our next story, learned a lot from asking himself the Love question during sex with his partner.

If I loved myself, how would I treat my penis/ vagina now?

Expectations and ejaculations

Nyall comes for help because he tends to ejaculate much sooner than either he or his partner want. As we start to look at what's going on within him during sex, it becomes clear that he's putting himself under tremendous pressure to perform. During foreplay he concentrates on 'getting it right' for his girlfriend. During intercourse his main focus is on doing it 'right'—and he keeps getting it 'wrong' by orgasming too quickly and disappointing his partner. Knowing he's likely to fail makes him a nervous wreck at the point of intercourse, which makes him even less able to exert control when he wants to.

What's very obvious is that Nyall is so focused on external factors—his girlfriend, his performance—that he isn't present to his own personal involvement in the sexual connection. He isn't experiencing intimacy with his girlfriend *or* with himself. Sex for him is like an exam—along with all the expected tension.

So we start working with the Love question. Along with answers to the Love question itself come the answers as to why this problem is happening. In Nyall's case, his self-loving answers to the dilemma of premature ejaculation show him that he has a pattern of feeling not good enough and trying to please others. He starts to see how much it's hindering his success in most areas of his life. His problem in sex is a gift in disguise.

Difficulties that show up in our sex life often reflect fundamental issues in our life in general.

The task we set is to use the Love question each time he begins to feel that familiar sense of pressure or stress during foreplay and sex. He finds it revelatory. His answers revolve around being less critical and being kinder to himself, and allowing himself to be in the moment: *If I loved myself, I'd focus on the feel of her skin under my hand/ I'd know I'm enough as I am/ I'd choose to relax/ I'd choose not to worry/ I'd know that I'm doing my best/ I'd know this isn't about performance but about her and me* … All this wisdom emerges from him in these fraught moments.

What also emerges is the realization that his girlfriend is very critical of him, which is why Nyall is so anxious to please her. Nyall starts to understand that sometimes he feels hurt and angry with his girlfriend—even during sex. His anxiety and difficulty in being fully present are partly because he feels judged. This Truth reveals itself when one answer to his Love question is: *If I loved myself, I wouldn't have sex with her now.*

Whereas Nyall thought he was dysfunctional and not good enough in bed, the answers to his question simply indicate that he isn't being true to himself during sex. The sex he's having is not self-loving. It's not intimate or connected—not with himself and not with his partner. When he starts to ask himself the Love question, he begins to hear his Truth, and it was ignoring his Truth that caused the problems. His girlfriend is not to blame—she's just being who she is. When Nyall starts to listen to himself, his response to his partner is more in line with what feels right for him, and their dynamic changes.

Nyall eventually ended the relationship, and is now with a woman with whom he feels completely safe and at home. His sexual 'problems' (the messages from his Truth) have mostly resolved—except when he puts pressure on himself. In other words, Nyall now loves himself more and listens to his Truth more regularly in his sexual life.

If you loved yourself, how would you handle expectations during sex?

When sex is painful

Pain during sex has a variety of possible causes. There may be a physical reason—if you experience pain during sex, please ask an appropriate doctor. Sometimes, however, the cause is not physical, and that's especially when the Love question can bring clarity. In Cassie's case, the answers she received to her Love question were surprising and life-altering.

Cassie has been married for five years, and sex with her husband is painful each and every time. She's learned to breathe through the pain, but while she enjoys the foreplay she's started to dread intercourse. She was a virgin when she married and expected to be able to have intercourse with her husband—she loves him, and wants to be with him in this way. She's surprised by the pain because she enjoys foreplay and thought she'd have no problem with sex. She has no history of sexual molestation of any kind, so there's no obvious trauma in this area.

We first check the physical aspects of her situation. She goes to a gynecologist and is declared organically normal and healthy. Then we begin to search for explanations. Her first time had been more painful than she'd expected, and we explore whether that initial experience might have set a precedent for her body to react with pain during intercourse, because the brain often takes the cue for future responses from a first encounter.

We explore how she feels about her role as a wife to see if resentments or expectations are getting in the way. We look at her parents' relationship and her schooling, and try to see if she's received guilt-inducing messages about women enjoying sex. We talk about her relationship to her body and how to improve her ability to feel pleasure and to be open, relaxed and intimate. In each of these areas we find something to understand and process. It's a rich journey, but the physical pain remains.

Cassie begins to ask herself silently during their love-making, *If I loved myself, what would I choose now?* and that's when things began to reveal themselves.

Her answers disturb her: *If I loved myself, I'd turn away from him now and make him stop touching me.* Initially she doesn't act on these Truths. They surprise, confuse and frighten her. After a while she can't ignore them and gently tries to honor herself without hurting or offending him. In our sessions she's distressed and seeks more insight: Why does she want to push him away?

As Cassie looks more closely, she begins to notice that her relationship with her husband is not what she's been telling herself it is. She begins to see that he doesn't act in trustworthy ways: he always has excuses for why he hasn't paid the bills, she finds out he's been chatting to other women online since before they were married, he doesn't support her as a partner and is an absent father to their children. She begins to understand that on some level she doesn't trust her husband. It's frightening to see things she's previously tried to ignore, but she finally understands it's causing her pain to allow him into her space, into her body and to be open and vulnerable to him in the way sex intends. Her body has been trying to tell her what her mind was unwilling to see.

Listening to her Truth liberated Cassie from living out a falsehood. It wasn't easy to see her Truth, but she preferred it to the alternative. What did she do? She listened to her heart's wisdom of what to do next and followed its guidance.

If I loved myself, what message from my sexual Self would I listen to now?

CHECK IN

How do you feel about you and sex right now compared with the start of this chapter? Has anything changed in how you view sex? Say something kind to your body right now. Then keep reading. Try to do this a few times throughout this chapter. By the end you and sex may have become closer friends.

Sex to avoid feelings

"I know I'm a sex addict," Donald tells me in our session. "I use sex to feel nurtured and cared for, but once it's over I want to get away from whomever I just had sex with. I feel trapped. But then I can't stay away for long—I need that closeness and love. I especially need it when I feel bad or something makes me feel unsure about myself. Then the craving gets so bad, I can't think clearly. I'll have sex with anyone who'll have me. Afterwards, I regret it. I know I'm hurting people. I can't trust myself. I manipulate men and women—I know what to do to make them open to me. I'm proud of that on the one hand, and hate myself for it on the other. I value honesty, but I'm not being honest."

He wants intimacy and can be physically intimate for a brief time, but when he has to show up as a person, the exposure feels dangerous and he has to flee. His eyes plead with me to understand and help him out of this vice he feels powerless to control.

This very sensitive, touch-hungry boy grew up in a strict, unemotional family. When something in his current life triggers the lack of holding and affirmation of worth he felt from his parents, he seeks out sex to avoid feeling the pain of that unmet need. After his need for feeling desirable and loved is sated, he faces having to engage with a real person. His experiences of engagement with his family were so painfully unsatisfying that it feels dangerous to his well-being to try it again. Hence the sprint for the door after sex.

We work with his self-love and affirmation. After a while he begins to ask himself the Love question before, during and after sex. He comes to his sessions in amazement.

"I realized if I loved myself, I wouldn't keep having sex with different people," he tells me with wide eyes one day. "It makes me feel very bad about myself and I'm left feeling emptier after."

Another day he understood he wants the cuddling more than the sex—he's just providing sex to fulfill the other's expectation. Still later, he sees it's the admiring and approving gaze he's after even more than the physical connection.

After a while he begins to work on affirming himself and asking himself the Love question any time he feels uncertain about himself or needy in some way. "I quite like myself," he says shyly one happy day. "If I loved myself, I'd keep remembering that. I don't need others to love me physically—that's just distraction. I need to love myself. I'm the real deal."

He still sleeps with anyone who's willing when he feels insecure, but he's becoming less tolerant of his own deceptions. "I don't lie to them anymore —I can't believe how direct I am sometimes. They must make their own choices. I can't be responsible for them like that. But I am responsible for telling my Truth." He feels at ease with himself more often. He still has to manage the cravings that come when he avoids meeting his real needs or feeling his feelings. Over time he's becoming more of the man he'd like to be. While the path is long and winding, he's following his Truth home to himself.

Do you ever use sex to avoid uncomfortable feelings?

If you loved yourself, what would you choose to do with those feelings now?

 Pause now, take a breath and say something kind to yourself

Listening to your Truth every step of the way

Our Truth doesn't always follow conventional paths.

You're the only one who can see your path and know your deeper needs and Truth. Following it feels good.

In the next example, Shari follows her path to unusual places with surprising results.

Shari has very little sexual experience and it affects her confidence with men. When she asks herself the Love question, her answer is: "I'd have random sex to practise more." Feeling good and self-loving in this decision she goes online, gets notifications from men wanting to 'hook up' and heads off to meet them and have (safe) sex. She feels pleased with her own courage but finds she doesn't really enjoy most of these encounters. She often feels nervous of the stranger and what might await her, and while random sex feels fun and interesting, it quite quickly becomes unsatisfying.

Shari achieved her goal—to ease her anxiety about her lack of sexual experience. Now she sees that it's no longer self-loving to continue what was self-loving to begin with. She decides her next step is to listen to herself better during sex. This results in her having such an intimate, open-hearted encounter with a one-night stand that they both feel deeply changed for the better by their mutual experience. Her needs keep changing, and she needs to keep listening.

If you loved yourself, what choices would you make about your sex life now?

Using sex to feel love

Emma is a beautiful, intelligent, gifted young woman in her early twenties, and when she tells me about her sex life I want to weep. Not because it's gruesome or abusive or shocking in any way—what makes me so sad is how she so chronically ignores her own needs. She behaves as though her voice, her opinion, her desires are completely irrelevant. She often sleeps with men she feels unsafe with—"But that's guys, right?"—and when she feels revulsion or reluctance, she finds reasons to convince herself to do it anyway. Surprisingly for her—but not for me—she often has bladder infections, thrush and bouts of depression.

Getting her to use the Love question is a long and difficult journey.

"If I loved myself?" she challenges me. "But what *is* love anyway? What does it mean to love yourself? Sure if I loved myself, I wouldn't sleep with them, but then who would I sleep with? If I was brutally honest, I'd say sex is revolting. It's only a way to get close to someone anyway. Guys like it, obviously, but they just get their kicks and then they can calm down enough to be close with you for a while."

For Emma, asking herself what she would choose if she loved herself is painful. It makes her aware of her own thoughts and feelings, and she has to face truths she's been trying to ignore. What it all boils down to is that in her life she's never felt she had a say in what happens to her emotionally. Sex is one place where she's found a sense of control. If she sleeps with a man, she gets some 'love' for a while—and she wants to feel love.

Why does she so badly want to feel love from a man? Because she doesn't live in an internally loving world, so she thinks love is only available to her from outside. She thinks sex is the only way to meet her needs for love and connection. Emma's life experiences have taught her these beliefs and her task is to learn to love herself. A cliché maybe, but then clichés only exist because they're true for so many people.

Whatever our personal histories, our task is the same: to learn to love ourselves and listen to our Truth, no matter what.

Emma is slowly becoming less afraid of the answers she receives to her self-loving questions. It's becoming less "impossible" for her to follow her Truth. She feels a little braver to hear it than before. One day she triumphantly tells me, "I stopped having sex with some guy right in the middle of it the other night. It wasn't making me feel good."

I almost cheer with excitement at this achievement. She's listened to herself and honored her Truth in a very real way. Question by question, she's finding her way back home to her Self, and she's learning to listen to her own needs.

Do you ever use sex to feel loved, even if you have to override your Truth?

If you loved yourself, how would you choose to engage with sex now?

The next section explains how to be true to yourself during sex.

Feel the feelings and meet your needs during love-making

When we're making love, the intimacy stirs a lot of feelings—some pleasant, while others (like anger, fear or sadness) can feel incongruous to sex. We usually try to turn away from these uncomfortable feelings and bring ourselves back to the task at hand. That's a sneaky way of not listening to ourselves in this most intimate of spaces.

Remember that feelings notify us about the state of our needs—for example, sadness may show us an area where we need tenderness. Avoiding the sadness doesn't allow the tenderness, and so you're blocked from the next level of intimacy and pleasure.

Knowing that your needs are expressing themselves to you, welcome *all* your feelings during love-making.

EXERCISE: FIGHT OFF NOTHING

If sadness, anger, fear or any other emotion arises while you're engaging sexually, know that these are parts of You saying hello. If you have an understanding partner, ask to pause so you can honor those feelings and see what you need to do.

Ask yourself the Love question at this time: your answer may be that you need to reassure yourself, cry, express something or ask your partner to hold you. This is all part of Truth in love-making. This is you being real.

If you feel your partner won't be open to such an honest expression of your needs, practice quietly inside yourself. Ask yourself the Love question and do your best to honor what you really need in that moment. Allow *all* of you to be seen and loved—at least by you.

Allowing yourself to honor your needs can increase your intimacy and pleasure immensely. Often, after feeling the feeling and acknowledging the need, your sense of intensity and pleasure escalate because your heart is more open to yourself and your partner.

What about sex and violation?

In a chapter about sex and love, I'd be remiss not to talk about difficult things like experiences of rape, molestation or too-early exposure to sex. These can be huge blocks to listening to your Truth and loving yourself. Experiencing sexual inappropriateness, hurt or attack raises questions such as: *How can I feel safe in the world and love myself if such bad things can happen? How can I open into my senses and sexuality again?* After experiences where you feel powerless to feel safe and happy in the world, you might say, "What's the point of knowing my Truth? It's too painful to acknowledge it and have it overridden—better to avoid my Truth and feel less pain".

Here's an analogy I find helpful with trauma.

> **THE RIVER**
>
> Picture a large, flowing river. In the river, scattered here and there, are big and small boulders that stick out of the water. In some areas there seem to be more rocks than water, yet the water continues to flow.
> A river flows around rocks and through difficult areas. The flow of a river isn't stopped by anything. Yes, it can be somewhat dammed up, but it cannot be stopped. It will flow and flow.
> You are this river. You exist and you flow all the time. When something painful or difficult happens, a boulder, or a whole lot of boulders, are placed in your life but you don't stop being a river.

In times of trauma or shock, we have inbuilt defense systems that help us survive. One of these is to prepare to die. If something truly awful happens and we think we might die, parts of us start to let go of life, and of ourselves, in preparation for no longer existing in our body. These parts believe we can no longer exist in the face of this event. Afterwards, even though we're physically alive, those parts that accepted death can stay in a shut-down mode. They remain that way until something happens to wake them up or until we deliberately bring them the message that they can return to life.

In trauma, rape, sexual molestation, sexual shaming, and too-early and/or shocking exposure to sexual content (for example, seeing porn as a child, walking in on someone having sex, being flirted with too young), whether it's a once-off, minor event or long-term, insidious abuse, a person may feel their sexual self has died or frozen up somewhat. In particular, they might feel they no longer have permission to exist as a sexual being, or they might not feel safe to enjoy, be present or listen to their own needs during sex. This part of them stays stuck at the boulder in the river, staring at it and grieving for what is lost, believing they can no longer flow.

While this can be a normal response, it's not accurate.

No matter what has happened to you, you don't lose your right to listen to your Truth or love yourself.

The river that is the real You continues to flow. No boulder can stop you from flowing, no matter what. You don't stop existing because something awful happened to you. 'Checking out' of being present is a normal response to trauma—however it can make the experience more horrifying because you feel alone in an awful situation. The pain and horror felt can also be responses to being abandoned by ourselves in this difficult circumstance. You're not there with you and this in itself is a kind of death.

Whatever your relation to your sexuality and body, asking the Love question—even in the direst of circumstances—can bring you closer to an internal experience of safety and love.

In that way, even the inner experience of violation can be mediated. The experience of the event is likely to be less traumatic if you don't feel like you die in it—not emotionally, not sexually and not spiritually. You know you are a river. You keep flowing.

 Pause now, take a breath and say something kind to yourself

Even in the midst of a trauma you can check in with yourself with the Love question. In any moment, you can ask, "If I loved myself, what would I choose to do now?" Your Truth in these hardest of moments can be as simple and surprising as at any other time.

> **SELF-LOVING INNER DIALOG DURING TRAUMA**
>
> - If I loved myself, I would know this is not my fault. I didn't want this. This person is violating my body but I'm still here. I still love me. I'll soothe myself now—I'll heal later. I'm still here. I still love me. This is not my fault. I have nothing to feel guilty or ashamed about. I'll just wait for it to be over and do what I need to survive. I'll be fine. I can still have my sexuality after this—it's mine and it can't be taken away from me.
> - If I loved myself, I'd let myself exist. I'd feel my feelings. I wouldn't take away my own future pleasure just because someone else didn't love themselves and took out their anguish on me.
> - If I loved myself, I'd still be me.
> - If I loved myself, I'd love my body even more now that this has happened to it because my body needs even more soothing love.
> - If I loved myself, I wouldn't be afraid. I'm here with me and I'll do what I need at every moment.
> - If I loved myself, I wouldn't blame myself for other people's choices.

If you feel you've 'died' even a little in your sexuality because of early, shameful or violating exposure to sex, it doesn't mean you've stopped being a river. You are a beautiful flowing river, and so is your healthy sexuality.

Every moment you listen to your Truth, you validate your worth and your existence. Every time you listen to your Truth and honor one of your needs, you love yourself back to life.

"In Your Self" has more tools to love yourself through shame, guilt and trauma.

If you loved yourself, what parts of yourself would you allow to flow more freely now?

Let yourself be loved

Stella has wanted to connect more with her body and her sexuality.

When we speak about it she says, "My wife touches me but I can't really feel any reaction. Even my breasts or vagina—it's nice enough, it's *OK*, but mostly I could take it or leave it. I feel like my body and me are two separate things. It makes me so unhappy. She loves me so much and she loves touching me and having sex—and there I am, like a zombie. I feel like I'm broken—like my system is faulty. I try to be present and feel it, but I have to concentrate so hard just to let myself focus on how it feels. I'm so busy trying to focus I can't relax. When I do succeed in concentrating on myself, after a while I feel disconnected from *her*. It's so hard for me! At the same time, I'm so busy worrying that she's OK and enjoying herself that I lose myself again. I'm 'in my head'—and this is supposed to be a body thing!"

One day she comes in with a big smile.

"I was with my wife in bed the other night," she tells me, "and I found myself feeling disconnected from my body again like I usually do. So I asked myself the Love question, 'If I loved myself, what would I choose now?' and the answer that came was, 'I'd let myself be loved.' It was such a revelation—I've never thought about it as letting myself be loved or not. It was amazing! I gave myself permission to be loved by her, and I was able to be connected and present with her and with myself, and I could *feel* my body's reactions and it was so heart-centered … Oh, it was just lovely. I did keep flitting in and out of my usual head thoughts, but I kept reminding myself over and over, 'Just allow yourself to be loved.' It wasn't perfect, it still took me ages to orgasm and I didn't manage to stay present and open the whole way through—the familiar frustration—but it was *way* better than before. Afterwards, and even now, there's this happy glow of love and connection. I feel hopeful and joyful. It's funny how asking myself if *I* loved myself, led to me allowing *her* to love me. Like only if I love myself can I let myself be loved by others. I know people say that all the time, but this is the first time I kind of understand it."

If you loved yourself, what would you allow for yourself now?

END OF CHAPTER CHECK IN

- How do you feel about sex in your life after reading this chapter?
- Has your view of your penis or vagina changed in any way?
- What would you like to say to yourself about your body and your sexuality?
- Is there any decision you'd like to make at this time about you and sex?

Watch the meditation video again or read the chapter summary to help you clarify your views. Write down your intention for yourself and your sexuality. You can use the chapter summary for this.

Here's the one-page summary of this chapter to download now to remind yourself of the key points of loving yourself in sex.

DOWNLOAD Chapter 8 summary
www.ifilovedmyself.com/members/chapter-8

Chapter 9

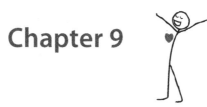

If I loved myself in my Parenting

The best that a parent can be is a demonstrator: A consistent, constant demonstrator of being in your own well-being.
Esther Hicks / Abraham

> **READ THIS CHAPTER EVEN IF YOU'RE NOT A PARENT**
>
> This chapter is about challenging relationships and why we become triggered and act in ways we wish we didn't—so it's relevant to everyone. If you're not a parent I suggest that as you read this chapter you:
> - replace the word 'children' with a person or situation that really triggers you (your work, family, colleague, money, body…); and
> - think back to your childhood, being a child of your parents or caretakers, and how they dealt with being triggered.

IF YOU LOVED YOURSELF, WHAT WOULD YOU DO NOW?

SET AN INTENTION FOR THIS CHAPTER NOW

Setting an intention is a powerful way of increasing the effectiveness of what you are doing. What do you want to get out of reading this chapter? Your intention is about your own needs and desired outcomes; it's unique to you and where you are in your life right now. Examples are:

- My intention while reading this chapter is to see and understand my patterns and choices that don't serve me in my parenting (challenging relationships) and how I might do things differently
- I have the intention to love and value myself in my parenting / relationships
- I intend to learn how to meet my needs more while I'm helping others.

Before you work through the chapter, scan this code to join me for a short video meditation about setting an intention for yourself and your relationships / parenting.

You can also access the meditation through this link: **www.ifilovedmyself.com/members/chapter-9**

It's all about needs

Parenting is one of the more intense areas to practice self-love—it's like self-love under fire.

Expectations, emotions and needs come at you constantly from surprising directions, and your reactions have real implications for the human beings who're dependent on you. I find my children have the capacity to trigger my big emotions and needs like little else. Sometimes those emotions are warm and cuddly and my needs are satisfied but other times ... they're not.

The point of loving ourselves is to meet our needs and live full and satisfying lives. The point of parenting a child is to meet their needs for the same reasons.

Like all humans, children have a long list of needs: they require food, shelter and education to survive and thrive, and they need safety, love, support, reassurance, acknowledgement and a whole host of other things for their optimum satisfaction and development. When we can meet our child's needs, all is well. When we don't manage that, things become difficult.

A friend once said to me, "You're only as happy as your unhappiest child." At the time I laughed, but since then I've noticed that the family's level of contentment really is affected by how OK the children are. When one of the children starts to express dissatisfaction with something, it can dampen everyone's good mood.

Unlike adults, children can't take full responsibility for meeting their own needs. They're still learning about what satisfies them, and they become overwhelmed by their negative feelings that indicate when a need is unmet. They really just *feel* fear or anger, and express it. It's the adult's responsibility to figure out which need is triggering those feelings. Is the child too hot? Scared? Hungry? Needing a hug? Needing something explained? By observing the adult's acknowledgement and meeting of their needs for them, children slowly learn to do this for themselves. Eventually they can say, "I need a hug/ Can you please explain this to me?/ I need attention/ I'm hungry." They also learn to love and reassure themselves as needed.

If no one shows them how to figure out what need a bad feeling is pointing to and how to care for it, they never learn to do it. They remain stuck in their bad feeling, expressing it with more and more intensity, waiting for someone or something to rescue them from how they feel. Many adults were never shown how to appropriately meet their own needs, and so are still stuck in that phase: overwhelmed when they feel bad, and looking for something external to make them feel better. That's where addictions often come in.

A problem faces us when we didn't learn this skill as children ourselves—we don't know how to look after our own needs—yet we have to teach it to our own children. So your child is overwhelmed when he feels big feelings—and so are you. Then there are two children—one big, one small—standing together scared or angry and feeling helpless. Those are the moments parents shout, shame, tantrum, threaten, punish, withdraw in a sulk ... We behave like children when our own childhood needs are calling for attention and we don't know how to soothe them. Don't worry, help is at hand!

Parenting is where you get to master skills you missed out on as a child—that's the self-love gift parenting offers.

When you feel overwhelmed by unpleasant feelings relating to your child (or anyone else), you get to see exactly where you lack the self-care skills you need. Next time you have a big emotional reaction to your child (or other), know that in this moment your own unmet needs are resonating with theirs. Instead of trying to make yourself feel better by controlling their behavior or blaming them for how you feel, ask yourself, "What do I need right now?

What's calling out for help within me? If I loved myself, what would I say to myself now? What would make me feel safer/ loved/ important/ cared for?" Then *take care of your need* while *caring for your child's needs*. I did warn you this was high-level stuff.

 Pause now, take a breath and say something kind to yourself

As your child goes through the different stages of development and you help to meet his or her needs, your own unmet needs from those stages make themselves known to you.

This is also what happened to your parents while they parented you. It can feel overwhelming and scary for a parent, but it's also a gift: a chance to finally love yourself exactly the way you once needed. Knowing this can turn the tough times into exciting opportunities—not easy, but at least more welcome. Keep reading—in the next few sections you'll learn how to do this. By the end of this chapter you might even find yourself deliberately seeking out parenting (or other interpersonal) challenges so you can love yourself even more!

- What needs of yours is your child or situation reflecting to you now?
- What needs do you think you reflected to your own parents?
- Did your own parents ever behave like children when emotions and needs were intense?

If you loved yourself, how would you start meeting your needs now?

Love yourself while parenting

Being responsible for a child is a great practice ground for listening to your own Truth and loving yourself well. Listening to yourself isn't easy in the constant bombardment of opinions from doctors, magazines, blogs and websites. Society puts a lot of pressure on parents to 'get it right', but the 'expert' suggestions may not meet *your* family's needs. Trying to follow advice that doesn't meet your needs can feel very disheartening. Following your own inner guidance might be a challenge, but it's much more satisfying. Did your parents follow their own Truth in raising you or did they follow what was socially expected? What did you learn from their example?

At any of the million daily decision points of what to do for your child, ask yourself the question, "If I loved myself, what would I choose to do now?" That's your most relevant, accurate and important guide.

Aim to feel loved in your childcare choices. That's all.

I could end this chapter here—except that learning to love yourself through parenting occasionally resembles a self-love boot-camp. The real training in self-love happens in those intense moments. You know what I mean: the moments where you, your child, both of you or the whole family are shouting, wailing or withdrawing, and you feel like you're about to explode with unmet needs, pain and not knowing what to do.

In parenting, the places where you don't love yourself enough rear up and tantrum at you. They throw up on you, keep you awake, drive you to distraction, terrify you, whine at you, elicit waves of sudden uncontrollable rage, make you crumple to the floor in a sobbing heap … In other words, you get to see your unmet needs through your reactions to your children.

Any reaction you have to your child is simply a reflection of how well your needs are met in that moment.

This is what was happening when your own parents had big reactions to you. When we love ourselves, we're compassionate and kind about our needs and feelings. When you feel calm and open-hearted towards your child, you can know all is well within you; your needs in that area are being sufficiently met. If you feel intense emotions about your child or their behavior, it's showing you a part of yourself that needs some loving attention and affirmation. If you can remember that, you'll feel a lot better in those overwhelming moments that seem to string together to make up the experience of parenting. It can also help you lean more openly and frequently into those wonderful, chest-swelling moments in which you gaze at those soft, rounded (or newly pimpled) cheeks and feel love chiming through your whole being.

If I look at my child as something I'm supposed to manage and control, I feel immediately overwhelmed. Why? Because we *can't* control anything outside of ourselves. More particularly, we can't control other people. Not even our children—not their behavior or their motivations or feelings.

Love yourself *more* when you feel bad.

When you feel irritated or angry with your child (or other), it's not really because of them. It's because something about their behavior—or the situation you find yourself in—triggers a previous experience you've had that relates to why you don't love yourself wholly now. I'll explain why this happens in the next section. Your reaction is actually just an indicator, a symptom of an underlying cause. The same way your body uses physical symptoms to highlight an area in which your self-love is not flowing freely, big negative reactions to your child's (or anyone else's) behavior indicate areas within yourself in which your self-love is not flowing freely. Let's look at *why* this happens.

If you loved yourself, how would you look at your reactions to your child now?

Why we get triggered

Let's use Mary to demonstrate how someone's behavior can cause a big reaction by dredging up old, well-hidden hurts we're unconsciously trying to avoid. Mary immediately feels irritated when a child is needy which indicates it's very likely she has some past hurt connected to a child being needy. All children are needy—that's their design—but not everyone has a problem with it. Mary's reaction to the child shows how *she* feels about what's being reflected about *herself*.

If Mary wants to change her automatic reaction of irritation, she needs to figure out what's triggering her. She can ask herself these questions:

EXERCISE: WHY DOES THIS TRIGGER ME?

- What do I feel when the child (or other) does that?
- What part of what s/he does really bugs me?
- If I could give my feelings words and let them speak uncensored—without judgment—what is the Truth of how I feel when s/he does that thing?

Mary's honest thoughts might be politically incorrect, for example: *This child is so irritating and whiny. I don't like her at all. I don't even know what she wants from me, but it feels like too much! I'd just hit her if I could—but I know that's wrong. I feel really bad that I'm thinking these things, but I wish she'd just go away. I can't handle her.*

Maybe you're thinking Mary sounds horrible but if you can see that (without realizing it) Mary is talking about herself, *then* how does it sound? Read it again.

Sad, isn't it? Our default programming is to treat ourselves as others have treated us in the past. From Mary's honest thoughts, it appears that somewhere in her childhood, she had needs that felt too much for someone. That person or those people couldn't handle Mary's needs, so she understood that her needs were too much for anyone—including herself—to handle. That's a very painful thing to feel.

We humans don't like pain—we push it away and get angry with things that cause it. So Mary has learned to respond with anger to her needy part (which never *did* get what she needed). And she does the same thing now. If she feels needy or is faced with a child who is needy, it reminds her of her own pain, and she gets angry with whatever she perceives is causing her pain—which is often the needy child.

Knowledge is power. When we know, we can choose. Once Mary has this knowledge about herself, she can see where it comes from and she can choose:

- to carry on judging, punishing and pushing away the child part of herself that didn't get her needs met. This way she'll continue to not meet her *own* deeper needs, for example, for acceptance and care. It also means she'll continue to take out her pain on children by pushing away *their* neediness; or
- to love and heal her own younger Self that's stuck in the painful belief that her needs are too much for anyone to handle—because it's not true. She can do that by identifying and meeting her real needs.

Children (and other relationships) bring you a whole lot of knowledge about yourself—whether you like it or not. And knowledge is power. So, next time you're triggered and out of control, behave in revolting ways and think horrid, unmentionable things about your sweet little darlings, remember that those shameful times can actually help you heal—depending on what you do with the knowledge they reveal about you.

What did your own parents do with the knowledge that raising you stirred in them? How did they respond to being triggered? What did you learn to do with your own feelings through their example?

If you loved yourself, what would you do with the things your children show you about yourself?

> **CHECK IN**
>
> How do you feel about parenting (and other challenging relationships or situations) right now compared with at the start of this chapter? Has anything changed in how you view the challenges of parenting? Say something kind to yourself right now. Then keep reading. Try to do this a few times throughout this chapter. By the end you and parenting (and challenging relationships or situations) may have become closer friends.

Use parenting to love yourself more

Being a parent is amazing for our individual growth. In my own life, my intention is to grow into more of my true self and live consciously and mindfully. This doesn't mean walking around calm and Zen all the time. It means being open to seeing myself, and learning to love and accept all of what I see—even when I see things I want to improve.

IF I LOVED MYSELF IN MY PARENTING

My children, for example, challenge the heck out of me daily and make me see myself in all my un-glory. Every day as they reflect back to me both my great worth and my deficiencies, I get to see myself more clearly—whether I like it or not. I'm grateful for this because I don't *want* any more 'heck' in me—as far as I'm concerned, they can go ahead and challenge it right out!

The way our society views parenting is very shaming and doesn't foster self-love. Parents are blamed for everything that goes wrong with a child. We're constantly bombarded with messages that we've failed if we don't get them reading early/ listening to classical music in the womb/ eating the perfect diet; that our children will be an embarrassment to us—a reflection of our inadequacy as a person. I don't see how this is helpful—except to the companies making money by selling us stuff to 'get it right'.

I find that using parenting as my own inner workshop—as opposed to thinking of it as something I'm supposed to 'get right'—is far more joy- and health-inducing. I don't feel as much pressure to be 'perfect', or like anyone else. My children are allowed to be who they are without huge pressure to conform to someone else's version of 'perfect' (except mine, of course!). I can just be me, and get it wrong sometimes, and right other times, and learn from both. This way, my children and I learn that it's OK to be who we are and to make mistakes, explore and grow, all in the context of being loved and listening to our Truth.

If I look at parenting as an opportunity to learn to love myself, grow and heal, I can more easily accept myself—and when I accept myself, I'm a *much* nicer mommy. It also allows me to more readily accept and face the challenges my children bring me—from misbehavior, to learning difficulties to illness—because I can see that they're driving me nuts for my own good.

Yes, I did actually say that.

In those crazy parenting moments, we're learning patience, generosity or how to love ourselves through times of shame. Mostly, we're learning how to love ourselves and listen to our Truth—over, and over, and *over* again.

As I see it, parenting is like attending a looooong course titled 'Learn how to love yourself no matter what', in which you get to workshop all the life skills vital for inner peace and contentment. We pay good money for that sort of thing normally, but if you're a parent you've got it for free right now! Well, OK, maybe not for free, but you *were* already paying for clothes, food, schooling, activities ... so you may as well get more bang for your buck, right?

This is also true for any challenging relationship or situation—you're already in it, so you may as well use it to your deepest benefit.

If I loved myself, how would I choose to use parenting or my challenging situation to increase my self-love now?

Where do guilt and shame come from?

Guilt and shame are feelings many people walk around with. (These are discussed more in "In Your Self") When someone can't accept his or her own guilt and shame, they try to get rid of it by passing it on to others. When someone feels guilt or shame and interacts with a child, there's a chance the child will learn to feel the same way. Then the child will carry it and pass it on, and so the cycle continues. If your parents did this with you, you likely do this with your children or anyone you get close to. None of us do it on purpose. I want to show you how to break this cycle for the sake of parents, children (including ourselves because we're all someone's child) and our world. This is a huge topic but I'm going to try distilling it to its essence.

If someone makes you feel bad in some way, it might indicate that they feel bad about themselves.

We humans usually avoid uncomfortable feelings. It hurts when we question our own worth or we sense we've behaved out of integrity with our Truth, so we instinctively try to make those feelings go away. Very often, in dealing with a child (or employee, colleague or partner), bad feelings are elicited in response to something they did or didn't do. It's therefore very easy to look at the child (or whoever you're blaming) and decide: *She's the cause of my bad feeling. If she behaved better/ listened more/ cared, then I wouldn't have this unhappy feeling.* You inform her of this and she understands she's not good enough for you. She feels shame about herself and guilty for making you feel bad. That's how it works: your own shame about yourself or guilt about your behavior is passed on to the other. We do this with others in our lives—personally, inter-culturally and globally. You usually don't feel better afterwards, but you feel *justified*. You can legitimately allow yourself to move away from the bad feelings because it was *her* fault.

But you're fooling yourself. Those bad feelings were there before the child (or whoever) came along because you don't love yourself in that place, and the feelings will remain there until you learn to love that part of you. The next time the child (or anyone else) does something similar, you'll feel the same way and blame it on her again—although it was never hers to begin with. You probably got this bad feeling from an adult who passed it on to you, and that wasn't about you either. Meanwhile, the child learns to pass on her own uncomfortable feelings too ...

It's time to break the cycle.

Own your feelings and LOVE YOURSELF when you feel bad in any way.

Remember that feeling bad is only showing you that you have unmet needs. Don't throw them onto someone else—that's not loving to yourself. Rather look for how you can meet your real needs. Practice asking the Love question in tough moments so that you learn to love and accept yourself even as you look at yourself honestly and take full responsibility for your behavior. *That's* what we need to be teaching ourselves, others and our children. There's no place for guilt and shame in a world of love.

And *please* remember your manners: if you realize you've done something wrong to your child (or anyone else), go and say a heartfelt sorry.

You will teach them more humanity and compassion in that simple act of sincerely apologizing to them than in many other things you try to pass on with words. Honor the being your child is, just as you would another adult, and acknowledge when you were in the wrong. If you aren't sure about doing this, imagine how it would've felt if your parents had acknowledged and genuinely apologized for their hurtful actions to you.

Go have a real conversation with your child where you take responsibility for your part in any unpleasantness. Shandra's story is next and it will help you understand exactly how to walk through these tough moments with love.

If I loved myself, what would I choose to do next time my parent, child or other makes me feel 'bad'?

 Pause now, take a breath and say something kind to yourself

Parenting through your needs

Shandra was raised in a home where she and her siblings were shouted at and hit if they did something 'naughty'. Her parents seemed to take it personally if the children did anything they weren't supposed to. "Why are you such bad children? Why do you do this to me?" her mother would shout at them. Shandra remembers feeling very ashamed as her mother looked down at her in disappointment. She can't remember what exactly she did that was so bad though.

Now she has four children of her own and when they fight amongst themselves or don't listen to her, she instantly feels furious. She can't control herself and shouts and hits. Afterwards, she feels ashamed of her behavior. She wants to know what she can do to change how she reacts.

"I hated it when my parents did this to me, but now here I am doing it myself. When it happens, I feel so angry and so helpless. I can't control them. Then I hit or shout so they'll *listen* to me. Afterwards, I feel justified because they behaved badly and they deserved it. But when my anger clears, I feel awful. No one deserves that, and these are my *children*! I love them. I'm supposed to protect them, not hurt them. I can't love myself—I don't deserve it."

"What do you think you need in that moment" I ask as we discuss one incident.

"Need? Oh my gosh, I need to be calm!" she responds with despair.

I persevere. "What do you need in order to be calm?"

Shandra stops and thinks a while. "I'd feel calm if they listened to me. If I knew I had control. If I wasn't scared of what they might do next, and that my voice meant nothing."

I can hear a number of unmet needs in her statement. Remember that acting on our negative feelings is simply an unhelpful way of trying to meet our needs. It's far more helpful to identify the real needs and address them.

"Shandra," I venture, "it seems you have a need to be heard?"
"Yes, absolutely! I want to be heard when I speak. I feel invisible sometimes."
"So you have a need to be heard and seen? To be important to them."
"Yes!"
"You say you're nervous of not being able to control them and of what might happen. I wonder if you have a need for safety?"
"Oh my goodness, that would be good. If I knew nothing bad was going to happen from their behavior, I could relax."

I can see that as we identify her needs, she's feeling calmer and calmer. She's sitting in a more relaxed way and speaking with less pressure. It's amazing how soothing it is to just acknowledge our needs—even if they're not yet met.
"OK, so we see some of the needs you have, and those weren't met in that experience with your children?"
"No, not at all!"
"And if they'd been met, you think you would've felt calmer?"
"I'm sure it wouldn't have hurt so much."
"What could you say to yourself that would meet some of those needs now?" I ask.
"I guess that I know they listen to me because they're scared of me. I do see they hear my voice. I don't want them to be afraid of me though," she adds sadly. "I know I'm important to them because they show me all the time how much they love their mom. It might help if I could remember that during those crazy times."
"It seems to me that your need for safety needs to be addressed somehow for the other things to be less stressful. What could you tell yourself—or do—to engage with that?"

Shandra thinks a while. "I actually know my kids are quite hardy. I don't really think anything bad will happen to them. And I'm good in a crisis so if something *was* to happen. I'd deal with it quite well ... It doesn't take away the fear, but it makes it less."

"So, if you loved yourself, what would you say to yourself about the children?" I ask.

"I think I'd focus on remembering that they're not doing this *to me*. They're children who're just learning how to live in the world. It doesn't mean anything bad about me. I'd remind myself that they do love and listen to me, and I don't need to shout or be scary." She laughs and adds, "I think maybe when they act up I should just start saying to myself, 'I am safe, I am safe, I am safe ...'"

*

It'll take time for Shandra to train herself out of the behaviors she learned from her own parents, but she's doing it by loving herself, one need at a time. Recently she told me about an incident where she'd shouted at her children in desperation, "I have a need to feel *important*!"

They stopped and looked at her in confusion. One said, "But you *are* important," and Shandra replied, "I don't feel important when you don't listen to me." Then those four little souls clustered around her and hugged her.

"It was such sweetness," Shandra said. "I felt so proud of myself for saying what I needed instead of accusing them."

If you loved yourself, how would you acknowledge your needs in challenging moments with your children or anyone else?

There's nothing wrong with you

I have worked in the healing field for over twenty years. I've been privileged to walk the path of healing with many individuals and groups in hospitals, clinics and private practice. During this time, I've heard horrible and disturbing stories about what humans can do and experience. What I've learned from witnessing humans heal is that underneath all our shame and guilt, all our imperfections, bad behavior and insecurities, we are beautiful, glowing beings. All that other stuff happens when we forget that Truth.

Whatever you feel bad about isn't because you *are* bad or faulty. It's because somewhere along the line you received a message that you're not acceptable as you are. Your behavior is merely a reaction to that lie. The bottom line is that each of us needs love and acknowledgment. When we don't receive this, a part of us becomes scared that we're not good enough to be loved. We worry we're not important enough to be listened to or worthy of having our needs met. There's nothing more painful in all of our human existence than believing we're unlovable, worthless or unimportant. Nothing beats that hurt—not loss, not trauma, not *anything*. Just about every stuck point in someone's healing journey comes down to one of those insurmountable, painful beliefs. Ironically, they're not even ever true!

As people return to seeing themselves as whole and worthy, I witness the troubling stuff gently fall away. It's useful to remember that it doesn't feel good to be out of alignment with knowing you're OK. Whenever you don't feel good, it means you're out of alignment with your Truth—the Truth that you're inherently valuable and worthy of love. Anything in your life that makes you feel less than good is actually *helping* you become aware that you're straying from your Truth, and not meeting your needs.

This is where parenting children comes in because as much as they bring us love and joy in the deepest of ways, our children also make us feel bad *a lot*.

Bless their teaching hearts. They just come along and trigger us wherever we still hold a belief that we're unlovable or not enough. They reflect our unmet needs to us. Probably because parenting is such an intense experience of attending to their needs, we get to see our gaps in loving ourselves through the needs we find irritating or difficult to meet for them.

When they do something that touches on those spots, we get angry, we shout, we try to discipline, we withdraw our love and approval, we try to escape from their neediness ... But they're not actually doing anything wrong. And there's nothing wrong with *them* either. They're just showing us where we need healing. A lot depends on how we deal with those reminders from our children.

When you have a big reaction to your child (or anything else in your life), it indicates that you've been triggered somewhere you hold the belief you're anything less than wonderful and amazing. If you recall, that's not true—the beliefs that we're 'not enough' mostly come from our own childhood experiences, from things your parents or teachers told you, how people treated you, how your needs were or weren't met ...

Those beliefs are NOT TRUE. Am I saying this enough?

Bottom line: There is nothing wrong with you. When your children—or anything else—drives you nuts, it's because you forget that.

We behave in ways we later regret or feel ashamed of because in those moments we forget that we're essentially OK and we were trying to avoid hurt. Blaming or bad behavior is usually an unsuccessful attempt at meeting our needs—for peace, safety, affirmation, etc.

Children, and other challenging relationships, constantly help you remember your true, glorious nature. Thank them, thank them, *thank* them for challenging you so deeply and so often. Children are powerful guides along the path to your Truth. Whenever they make you feel bad feelings, they're actually helping you learn to feel better. In the moments you feel overwhelmed or bad or guilty, ask yourself the question, "If I loved myself, what would I choose to do now?" Then follow your Truth step by step back to your natural shining Self.

It's there, it really is. You wouldn't be reading this book if it wasn't.

 Pause now, take a breath and say something loving to yourself

Children help us hear ourselves

I want to share Alan's story to show how his daughter Hannah offers him profound healing. The important thing to know about Hannah is that she's just like Alan—and that freaks him out no end.

Alan lives with a terrible lack of permission to be himself. He's lived most of his life with a grey, scared, bored sort of feeling, and he doesn't prioritize his needs at all. Psychiatrists have called it chronic, treatment-resistant depression with anxiety features. I call it reactive depression, and I'd even go so far as to call it a lifestyle disease. If our main purpose in life is to become the fullest possible expression of ourselves, then not having permission to be yourself is a living death.

Alan's parents were both deeply unhappy people and his mother was very controlling. Like many children do, young Alan set himself the impossible task of making his parents OK, thus learning to shape himself to other people's desires. He never learned that it was OK to just be himself—quite the opposite, actually.

Alan, of course, married an unhappy, controlling, scary woman just like his mother. He gave in to her pressure to have children, and he often feels totally overwhelmed by them—in particular, his eldest daughter, Hannah, who is insecure, socially withdrawn, anxious and bored. Just like him. Hannah's problems are multiplied because she also struggles with a learning difficulty. She should actually be in a different school, but Alan's wife refuses to acknowledge this and he's been keeping quiet. As usual. But it's getting harder than usual to not speak out.

Alan *knows* how it feels to be Hannah, and not be accepted for who he is. To be forced to live a life that doesn't suit him. He sits in my treatment room in tears, face wracked with pain about what his daughter is going through. What can he do? Alan's life-long depression is a result of shutting down his needs to please other people. He's very afraid of showing his true Self. He does have his own view on things—he just hides it really well. He wasn't taught to love and value himself or his opinions. Now along comes Hannah, offering this healing.

Why healing? Well, from his dismal and overwhelmed reaction to her, he has been given these gifts:

1. He finally gets to see exactly how he felt as a child and what his needs were. Many of his self-beliefs were formed at a time when he wasn't aware that his parents' issues had nothing at all to do with him. Part of him still thinks their unhappiness was somehow his fault, and he can't love or trust himself because of this. He can, however, see that none of this is Hannah's fault.
2. He gets a chance for a do-over. This is his moment to finally speak out about what a child like this needs. It's an opportunity to honor himself—for his own sake, and for his daughter.

Author Sir Thomas Moore says depression is your soul calling you home. Alan's soul has been calling for most of his life, but he's never felt he was worth listening to. Will he find the courage to start listening now? This time, his life isn't the only one at stake. His daughter could also be his trigger for healing a lifelong pattern of repressing himself—if he's willing. In my opinion, his depression can lift if he is willing. And if he isn't, he has to watch her suffer—just like him. He's taking small, brave steps. My heart and soul are cheering him on.

Children make it harder for us to bear sufferings we've become used to. Something that's 'fine' for you is not so for your child. They bring us closer to hearing our soul. When you're faced with your child's struggle, ask yourself, "If I loved myself, what would I choose to do now," and follow the Truth you hear. Follow it tiny step by tiny step if you need to—that's the way mountains are climbed.

Parenting is not all hardship and suffering though! Let's look at some pleasant stuff now.

If you loved yourself, what would you choose to do now?

Let yourself love

One of the gifts of parenting is that you get to love and be loved by someone in an intimate, real, daily-life way that at the same time transcends all daily-life stuff. It's a bit mind-boggling to ponder one's relationship with one's child. There are so many angles and tones.

Who knows us as intimately as our child does? They see us at our best and at our worst, in public and in private, dressed and undressed, on stage and on the toilet. We see them when they're happy and when they're sick, we're their worst nightmare and their best fantasy, the source of their deprivation and their good things.

Most of the time we focus on the daily grind: feeding kids, dressing kids, getting kids' homework done, making sure kids' stuff is in kids' bags, coordinating lifts for kids and worrying about discipline/ how to get kids to listen better/ respect you more/ not hit their brother/ be a polite, upstanding member of society... There's the exhaustion of the non-stop picking up off the floor, chasing after them, washing dishes, making food (that they complain about), fielding "I'm boooored"/ "You're not the boss of me!"/ "Why can't I? All the other children are ..." Can you *believe* parents do this stuff every day?!

While I'm dancing the parenting dance, I try to also remember to sneak regular peeks into the core—the love between me and these beings that are my children. That love that's just as mind-boggling as the daily grind. Whether or not things are good between us, it's a pure, direct, unquestioned connection between my heart and theirs.

That kind of connection sounds lovely in theory but in reality it's something many of us avoid. (There's more on intimacy in "In Your Self") We feel vulnerable and exposed when we let ourselves be open, and I've found it requires courage to stay open to intimacy. I think maybe that's why so many of us spend most of our time focusing on the daily grind—it's exhausting, but it distracts us from our heart's wide-open vulnerability regarding our child. I've heard people say of their children, "It's like having your heart walking around in the world and you have no control over what happens to it." There aren't many of us who wouldn't protect ourselves from *that*. And we protect ourselves by shutting down our love a little—making it a *little* less vulnerable. So as parents we provide, we work, we 'do', but we avoid 'being' because it's too real and too raw for many of us. School holidays can raise anxiety—all that time together, all that potential intimacy ...

Life can become bland and meaningless when you're scared to add spice because you're worried it'll be overwhelming. Protecting yourself from love makes for a bland life. If you're ready to enjoy the flavors of your life, this is what I recommend:

EXERCISE: THE SWEETNESS OF LOVING

Gaze at your child (or loved one) and focus on the love you feel for him or her. Open your heart to whatever degree you're able in that moment and let yourself taste the sweetness of loving this child. It's never the same flavor: sometimes it's tinged with bitterness, at times with spice, sometimes it's a little sour, sometimes subtle, sometimes rich, sometimes overpoweringly sweet.

As you look at your child eating, getting ready for school, picking their nose, sitting reading, resisting what you're telling them, being rude, *whatever*, think about the fact that you really love this person. Let that be the main thought in your mind as you deal with them. Allow your heart to open. Sometimes you may look at how disgusting they're being and feel amazed that you love this child; at other times it'll be obvious that you do. Whatever the flavor, drink deeply from this love. It's always enriching, grounding and satisfying.

Use this exercise with yourself too. Every time you observe yourself in some way, allow your heart to open up to love for You. Add the spice of love to your life.

If I loved myself, how would I look at myself now?

Does your child frustrate you?

You know those times when you want your child to do something, and they just don't? You say it again, you get louder and more irritated. While the thing still isn't done, you feel anger and pain rising up in you—*Am I so unimportant that my child won't even do this thing I've asked of them which they* know *needs to be done?* You feel hurt and unloved and end up shouting, being rude, handling them too roughly or nagging.

Someone recently told me that her daughter said, "Mom, don't rash me all the time." 'Rash', you know, like something irritating on your skin—that's how it feels from their side. We're 'rashing' them. Just because we need to get things done, tidy the house, feed, fetch and carry …

Let's first have a look at *why* we might feel so frustrated at those times, and why children might resist what we ask of them. You might be surprised: it has to do with loving yourself and meeting your needs!

An adult and a child have very different takes on the world.

On the one hand, an adult can see *the overall picture*—the many balls we're juggling. It's our job to keep those fast-moving balls in the air, and to do this well we need some space to move in, right? If you need to suddenly lunge for a ball, you can't have a little person standing in the way—that'll throw you off your game. You'll drop a ball. You'll do it wrong. You'll fail. "No little people underfoot, please," is what we'd like to say. "You need to cooperate so I can do this right."

Your child, on the other hand, is involved with what's happening *in the moment: Ooh, this book/ hamster/ booger in my nose is right here, right now and I want to explore it. It's so interesting.* (A faint sound from beyond the realm of Right Here and Now brings only vague awareness.) *No, shhh– I'm very busy with this thing.* (Sink back into the dream state.) *Someone's calling.* (Awareness slowly rising from deep down.) *Huh? What's she saying? Get up? Brush my teeth and get ready for bed? Huh? No, no, no.* (Sink down again into the activity.) *Back to this—it's so rich. I don't want to stop and do that other thing—ugh! She's interrupting me!*

Even though *you* can see he needs sleep otherwise he'll be tired in the morning, to him morning is another planet. He's deeply involved with something—even if it doesn't look like anything 'worthwhile' to you.

Your child's reality and yours live side by side. You have your point of view, and your child has theirs. Both are valid. One thing is not more important than the other thing. If your child doesn't listen to you, it doesn't mean you're not loved or worthy. They don't need to make you feel OK—*you do*. Thank goodness for that because they're *so* inconsistent in their affirmations, aren't they? You, however, can choose how consistently you affirm your worth—and you do this by listening to yourself and following your Truth.

Rather than expressing anger at your child, you can identify and meet *your* needs. (You can use the list of needs on page 32 to identify what's going on for you and page 37 for how to feel your feelings.) Talk to *yourself* lovingly and reassuringly when you feel upset in any way. When you feel frustration or anger, ask yourself the Love question and listen for guidance. Your self-love voice knows what you really need—and how to best meet it.

IF I LOVED MYSELF IN MY PARENTING

If I loved myself, what would I choose to do now?

 Pause now, take a breath and say something kind to yourself

Love first, everything else second

Tanja comes to me in great distress. It's an impossible-seeming situation: her sixteen-year-old daughter has started smoking marijuana. She's skipping school, telling lies and not willing to talk to anyone in the family about anything. She's failed two school terms but she *could*—if she works hard—rescue the situation and maybe still pass the year.

They live in an impoverished neighborhood where drugs, truancy, gangs and illiteracy are high. Many people around them are unemployed but they're among the more fortunate—they live in their own home and Tanja is employed. While her salary is enough only for basic living standards, that's more than many of their neighbors have. Tanja sees her daughter hanging out with a group of boys she knows do drugs—she knows some of them smoke methamphetamines (tik)—and she's terrified of what might happen.

She wants her daughter to wake up and see what her choices might lead to. So far, Tanja tells me, she's shouted and pleaded. She's pulled the guilt card—"Look how much I've done for you. You're going to kill me because of my high blood pressure"—and threatened to throw her daughter out the house. Tanja is crying in the evenings, stressed out during the day and is really not OK—her daughter's life is in danger and she feels she has to take action. But how?

As we talk it through, I ask about her daughter's good traits. Tanja is quick to tell me that she's kind, considerate, bright, funny and ambitious. I can see her soften as we speak about the good stuff.

"Do you love her?" I want to know.

"Yes, of course," says Tanja.

"Have any of these good things about your daughter, or your love for her, gone?" I ask.

"No, it's still there under all this."

"Would you really want to kick her out of the house?" I ask gently. Tough love is very good at the right time, but in this case because it's the very start of the problem, it would put her daughter more at risk.

"No, not really. I just don't know what else to do. I'm so scared of what'll happen to her," Tanja says tearfully.

"Do you believe love is more powerful than fear?" I ask.

"Yes, definitely," she answers.

Slowly we turn our focus to the approach of love first, everything else second.

"How can love play a role here? When your mother loves and believes in you," I remind her, "that has a very deep impact. What if you told her something like, 'I see you as you are. I see your good, no matter what. I believe in you. You are wonderful and powerful, and you can do whatever you set your mind to.'"

We discuss how giving her daughter that message consistently—especially in a time where she's showing her 'bad' stuff—will inoculate her daughter a bit from seeking to meet her needs for love, approval and good feelings from questionable friends and substances. Tanja has to help her daughter learn to look inside for that love, and she needs to do that for herself too.

"Be her safe place," I suggest. "Don't make her safe place scary and rejecting. You do need to set boundaries and say when you're upset, but reject the behavior, not *her*. Let her have her life and make her choices—but keep reflecting those choices to her, affirming her worth and reminding her that she can choose other things for herself. She's facing difficult choices right now—choices she'll have to live with for the rest of her life. Remind her of that, and remind her that she's wonderful. Encourage her rather than accuse her. Love first, discipline and education after." Draw closer to her with love, rather than withdrawing as punishment.

All of this is seeping into Tanja's mind as we speak. I can see she's thoughtful, calmer and more hopeful. Her fear had led her to cut off her daughter emotionally, making her feel as though she'd already lost her, which frightened her further. Our conversation is reminding her of their bond. It's giving her daughter back to her.

I finally say, "If you loved yourself, what would you choose to do now? What would make you feel most at peace, happiest, proudest of yourself—not just for a moment, but for a long time after?"

Tanja is quiet a long while, and I can see that she's dropped deep into herself. Then she looks up with an expression of amazement.
"Oh, it's *my* journey. It's about *me* too. It's not just, 'How can I control her and the boys to make things the way I want them to be?'"

When Tanja left the room a short while later, she did so full of vigor and purpose.

Later she told me she had gone home and called all her children together to tell them she loves them and she's there for them. They responded well and things have become somewhat easier at home. "I'm so grateful for this", she tells me "In my culture we don't talk to children like this. But it's much nicer for me."

Her relief at having her power back was clear: If she loves herself, it seems she will remember to focus on her own journey. That way, she'll make clearer decisions about how to respond to her daughter's actions.

First love—for yourself and all those around you. Everything else after. Love yourself, then take action from that space of knowing who you are and loving yourself unconditionally.

If I loved myself, what would I choose to do now?

A QUICK CUPPA LOVE

Jay wrote this to me:
"I usually do a weekly shop on Monday and this Monday I felt I should do that, but my energy levels were so low. Then I asked myself the Love question and I thought about how I really didn't want to. I really just wanted a cup of tea and some quiet time while my son was sleeping, before school pick-up, ballet lifts, dinner prep, etc. And then I thought how, if I was advising a friend, I definitely wouldn't make her feel like she had to go to the shops—and yet I was about to do that to myself. So I looked in the freezer and found something OK for supper, and decided everything else could wait. I felt really good! And there was no negative comeback. In fact, it got me thinking about all the other times I haven't let myself off the hook because of wanting it to be all perfect and as planned."

If you loved yourself, what would you choose to do now?

Be gentle with yourself

When I tell people, "Be gentle with yourself," they sometimes look at me as though I'm speaking a foreign language. I suppose in a way I am. Treating ourselves kindly and gently is unfamiliar to a lot of us. We seem to have the idea that there's a 'right way' and anything other is 'not right'. When we don't get it 'right', we think we're not good enough. Thinking we're not good enough leads to all sorts of nastiness—low self-esteem, depression, addictions ... When it comes to parenting, many of us are very busy trying to get it 'right'— although, truthfully, none of us is quite certain what that means. How could we, with all the opinions out there?

This 'right way' thing is a very ungentle and self-destructive way to live. I was vividly reminded of this by my own little master teacher, who felt it necessary to give me an in vivo practicum. Here's what happened:

I was trying to meditate but my son, who was six or seven at the time, just wouldn't leave me alone. I asked him, told him, pleaded with him to just give me a few minutes on my own, but he wouldn't leave. He was truly magnificent in his persistence and determination, and I so desperately needed that space that, finally, I cracked. I slammed my way into the bathroom and SCREAMED in frustration. Just by myself, mind you, not at him. Even so, my wild banshee-like wail freaked him out and things went pear-shaped, with tears all round. I was so down on myself afterwards and I had a whole list of wrongs.

First, I hadn't kept my cool during meditation. I mean, I was *meditating*, for heaven's sake! But I'd allowed myself to get riled up, attached to the outcome I wanted and revealed that I'm no yogi yet. Very disappointing—I'd expected more from myself.
Second, I'd gotten angry and acted out my anger. Definitely not a yogi.
Third, I'd lost control. Yup, not enlightened.

Fourth, I'd frightened my child ... And on and on, deep into 'right way' territory.

When I brought my sorry story to someone who loves me, he laughed. "He pushed the boundaries big time! You went into the bathroom to scream. You didn't let it out at your child. You did your best to protect him from your anger, but he got to see it and feel it. Afterwards, you loved him and explained it to him. How could it be better? Do you want to raise your child thinking people always have their shit together? That *he* has to always hold himself together? How would that help him in the world? You showed him there are limits, that we all lose it sometimes, we all have big emotions and that it's OK. We apologize and make sure our connections are still intact."

What? It was actually *better* that I'd been so imperfect?

Hmmm ... That actually did make sense to me. Oh, what a relief—and thank goodness for confidants! I could see then that I'd done just fine.

So why had I been so hard on myself? If I'd been gentle with myself, I could've enjoyed the gift sooner. If I'd just loved myself or asked myself the Love question at any stage, it would either have calmed me down, or stopped my guilt and self-shaming sooner.

My tricksy little teacher had aided me in seeing (again) that the fantasy 'perfect' is not actually helpful. Neither is getting uptight about getting it 'wrong'. Whipping ourselves into shape is not showing love for ourselves. The reason it hurts so much is because when we follow 'perfect' or 'right', we don't listen to our Truth or our real needs.

Let me repeat that so we all hear and absorb it:

'Perfect' is a load of nonsense. It's *much* more effective to be gentle with ourselves. Be loving with You. You are just fine as you are.

Just ask, "If I loved myself, what would I choose to do now?" and follow what your heart tells you. *That* will be perfect. For you.

Love yourself as much as your child

When Nomsa was a child, her parents were mostly occupied with fighting each other. She was an only child and their shouting, arguments, depressions and cold wars dominated the house. If she needed help with something, it was difficult to get their full attention. If she looked for attention or love, she was usually disappointed. She learned to find her own comfort from playing with her dolls and later going out to friends' houses as much as possible.

Now she has a little girl of her own and she's finding it extremely difficult to manage the emotions that surge through her in response to her daughter, Noni. Not wanting to repeat her parents' behavior, Nomsa has made very sure that Noni has consistent love and attention, and can ask for what she needs. Noni feels so comfortable with this care that she expects it and— Nomsa feels—takes it for granted. Nomsa sometimes wants to shout at Noni for being a spoiled brat.

"What's the emotion you feel when that happens?" I ask.
"I'm not sure. I just know I feel like I can't handle it. Like I'm going to die or something. Something inside me wants to shut her *down*."
"If the feeling had words, what might it be saying?"

Nomsa thinks a moment and I remind her to let the feeling speak rather than her mind.

"It would say, 'Who do you think you are, little girl. Why do you think you get to have this nice stuff? I never had nice stuff. Why do you think you're so great? I hate you.' Oh my gosh!" She looks at me with round, scared eyes. "I'm a horrible person! How can I say that about my daughter? It's not even true, is it? I love her most in the world. I don't know what made me say that!"

"Is that how you felt as a girl? How old do you feel inside when you say that?" I ask gently.

Her eyes fill with tears. "I feel about four or five. I didn't get any of the love and attention she gets. Sometimes I can't understand how she doesn't see how good she has it. She just wants *more*. And I have to give more when I didn't even get it myself."

"So, the big feelings you feel, do you think they're the little You's feelings?"

"Yes, I think so. I remember feeling stupid for wanting my parents' attention. Like, who am I to think I deserve them turning to look at me. They were busy with their grown-up stuff. I'd just go quietly back to my room and try to pretend it didn't matter ... but I remember I'd get this horrible lumpy feeling in my throat. Then I'd play with my dolls, and make up stories where this doll was the most precious princess in the world, and everybody loved her, and no one could take their attention off her because she was so wonderful. Isn't that ironic?" Nomsa is quiet a while. "Now Noni is that princess, and sometimes I can't bear the unfairness of it. I want her to have it, but it hurts so much that I didn't get it. I think that's what the feeling is. I don't know what to do with all those big feelings inside me. I'm scared they might kill me or make me say something horrible to her."

"So, what do you actually need in those pain-filled moments when you just want to shout at her for feeling so worthy?" I want to know.

"I think I wish I had the confidence she has, and that I'd received that love."

"If you loved yourself in those moments, what would you choose to do?" I ask.

Nomsa's eyes again fill with tears and this time they overflow and make two shining stripes down her cheeks. "I'd tell myself, 'I am just as precious as this amazing little girl standing in front of me.' I'd say, 'See? This is how to know you're worth paying attention to: do it like her. Look how wonderful you are for creating her. I love you, Nomsa!'"

 Pause now, take a breath and say something kind to yourself

You are the voice in your child's head

I was in a group discussing the way we talk to ourselves. As people shared, it became apparent that the way we speak to ourselves is something we learned to do. As people opened up about how they talk to themselves, we noticed the critical tones most of us used: *Why did you do that?/ What will people think?/ That wasn't good enough./ No one will love you if you're like this.* For many of us, our self-talk was a running commentary on what we weren't doing well enough, combined with some mean scare tactics like, *If I don't do it right, then ...*

Someone commented that we talk to ourselves as though we're children, and this led to a realization that the way we talk to ourselves seems to mimic how we were spoken to as children. This suggests that when you're alone, your default inner voice is your parents' or caretakers' voice. Apparently—unless we make a specific effort to change it—no matter how old we are or how long it's been since we heard our parents or teachers, when we talk to ourselves, we use their voice and tone. Whether this is a good or horrible thought for you depends on the role your parents played, and what part of their message you took into your Self.

I had a beautiful example of this when my child was two years old. Back then he had a cautious approach to life, and was often scared to do physical things like climbing or swinging high. I'd encourage him, gently saying, "*You* can do it," in a sing-song voice. I only know it was a sing-song voice because one day we were at the play park, and I noticed him trying to climb up a ramp. I watched to see what he'd do, and I saw him falter, pause and consider going back down. And then he quietly said in a sing-song voice, "*You* can do it," and continued laboriously climbing till he'd made it to the top, where he looked really pleased with himself. As for me, I was completely thunderstruck by hearing him using my voice and words to encourage himself. He had integrated my message: I was the voice in his head.

Since this brazen demonstration, I've tried to make sure the messages I give my children will serve them for the rest of their lives. I know how the messages in *my* head have helped and harmed me, and I feel so blessed to have the magic power to give my own children good voices and messages *on purpose*.

Of course, I very often don't get it right. I hear myself in their conversations with each other. When one child speaks in short, sharp accusations to the other, I see myself too. Then I step into full hypocrite regalia and say in a short, sharp accusatory tone, "Don't speak to your brother that way!" Ah well, you can't win them all.

Consciousness is what we're after here: Be aware that you're building a human being, and your voice will be the guidance in their head in their most private moments.

What will your child hear in his mind when he faces a struggle or a disappointment? What voice will speak to her within when she needs courage?

What is the voice in your own head? If your inner voice is not as loving or encouraging as you'd like it to be, actively change it now. (More on how to do this in "In Your Self"). If your children are already grown up, it's not too late to use your Parent Magic for good. Even adults still listen to their parents' feedback with extra attention—you'll be amazed what a few positive words from you will do for your adult children.

Say loving and encouraging things to your child daily.

You won't spoil them: on the contrary, you'll build a human being who can love themselves. Our world really needs that.

Build yourself into that human being too. Say a nice thing to yourself each day, and see what happens to the voice in your head.

Oh, and *please* do me and the world a big favor and start teaching any children you know to *listen* to their *own* Truth. Ask them, "What feels right to you?" when they're not sure what to do. "What would the big loving part of you say to do now?" And ask yourself the same thing.

If you loved yourself, what inner voice would you choose for yourself and your children now?

IF YOU LOVED YOURSELF, WHAT WOULD YOU DO NOW?

> **END OF CHAPTER CHECK IN**
>
> - Do you see parenting in the same way as before this chapter?
> - What has changed?
> - How can you use parenting for your own self-love, growth and healing now?
> - Is there any decision you'd like to make at this time about something you find challenging in your parenting?
>
> Watch the video again or read the chapter summary to help you clarify your intentions. Write down your insights—perhaps on the chapter summary.

Here's the one-page summary of this chapter to download now to remind yourself of the key points of loving yourself in parenting.

> **DOWNLOAD** Chapter 9 summary
> www.ifilovedmyself.com/members/chapter-9

Conclusion

There's no wrong or right way to do life

All you need to do in your life is to be yourself.

Each of us is an expression of life.

You can't get an expression of life wrong. You just can't. You are the way you are because that's what *your* expression of Life looks and feels like. However you look, whatever you're able or unable to do, however grand or simple your life is, your task is to relax, make your daily choices based on what makes your heart sing sweetly and joyously and enjoy as much of your life experience as you can. Living your most satisfying life will inevitably benefit those around you—even if merely by inspiring them to listen to their own heart Truth.

That's it. The secret to a satisfying life.

Shine on

Now we come full circle to where we began: Arnan sitting on my couch in my psychotherapy practice, trembling with excitement on the precipice of fully living life as himself.

"I think our task in life is to become a full expression of ourselves," I comment. Arnan looks at me quizzically. "What do you mean?"

"Each one of us has to learn to allow ourselves to be whoever we are, fully and unashamedly. That's when we can all shine. That's when the world will be better."

He thinks a while and then says, "So you mean live to our edge?"

"Our edge?" I ask, wanting him to explain more. It sounds good to me, and the energy with which he says it feels liberating and exciting.

"Yes," he says. "Right now there's a gap between me and my edge." He shows me with his hands where his body ends and where he imagines his edge does, "You're saying live all the way to the edge?" He brings his inner hand towards the outer until they meet.

"Yes!" I say happily. "Your task is to close that gap, to expand into yourself all the way to the edge. When you give yourself permission to be yourself, you feel love for all that you are and you don't even consider apologizing for it."

Arnan closes his eyes and lets himself feel this concept quietly for a few moments. Then he suddenly bursts out laughing and, opening his eyes, exclaims, "What a relief!"

Isn't it just?

I happily anticipate the day he realizes there's no edge.

THE BEGINNING

Thank you for you

On behalf of myself, the Earth and all beings, I thank you deeply for intending to love yourself and listen to your Truth. My heart tells me this is how we will heal as a collective. I'm grateful for your presence here, for your unique shine, your piece of the greater puzzle. Thank you for all that you are and all that you do.

May you find love, joy and wholeness as you follow your Truth to your edge— and beyond ...

With love and light

Eilat

Work with me

If you'd like to work with me in person, I offer individual sessions, group sessions and workshops to help you and your community find your Truth and live it. I can also speak to your group or at your event.

You'll find the descriptions and details on my website.

www.ifilovedmyself.com/work-with-eilat

or contact me at:
info@ifilovedmyself.com

PART THREE

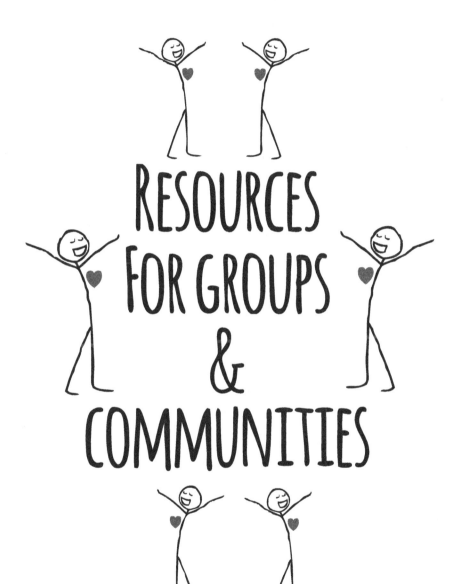

RESOURCES FOR GROUPS AND COMMUNITIES

The self-love revolution

Where two or more are gathered with one common goal of love, there is the presence of God.
Michael Mirdad

This is a great book to read as a group, family or company because as more of your community is empowered to listen to their Truth, a culture emerges of easily honoring each other's way in the world. It creates a safe, peaceful and productive space for you all.

Those who know me will tell you I encourage everyone around me to follow their heart's Truth. The more the merrier! They also deeply understand and support me when I do the same. The other day I bumped into a friend I hadn't seen in ages. She was dressed in gym clothes, clearly on her way to a class. We were so excited to see each other and wanted to catch up. We started chatting a mile a minute and she glanced at the time and said, "I really want to spend time with you now. I was going to gym but I guess I could skip it ..."

I could see she was torn between two things she really wanted to do. I responded, "If you loved yourself?"

She immediately straightened up, all signs of painful indecision gone. "I'm going to gym. Bye!" she called out and cheerfully jogged off down the road, leaving me laughing in delight.

My friends and family ask each other this question to support honest decision-making in every choice from diet to medical matters, family dynamics, parenting, career moves ... Making your decisions from your Truth leaves you feeling at peace and excited about yourself and your life. Who wouldn't want to live in an environment like that?

Three ideas for building a self-love community

1. Discuss the book with your friends, compare notes and agree to encourage each other to ask the Love question and listen to your Truth in your lives. You can also work through the book or workbook together.

2. Bring this to your existing group or book club or start a group which meets regularly; weekly, every two weeks or once a month. Download my supportive guidelines on how to structure a group as well as ideas for group conversations. You can work through the work book together as a group.

DOWNLOAD HOW TO STRUCTURE AND RUN A GROUP
www.ifilovedmyself.com/members/group-guidelines

3. Approach a leader in your community who you think may be interested in enhancing the supportive, productive and harmonious elements of community—your minister, boss, colleague, teacher, school principal, doctor, healer. Discuss the group benefits of bringing this ethos and the Love question into the daily functioning of your community. Download the free discussion points and ideas to consider.

DOWNLOAD HOW TO CREATE A SELF-LOVE COMMUNITY
www.ifilovedmyself.com/members/community-guidelines

Contact me at www.ifilovedmyself.com if I can help.

RESOURCES FOR GROUPS AND COMMUNITIES

One last thing

Please help me broadcast this message of self-love by leaving a review of this book on Amazon, Goodreads, Barnes & Noble, BookBub and any other online book community you know of. You'll really be helping me because reviews are an author's lifeblood nowadays. If no one reviews a book, it fades into the archives and no one can access it anymore. I really appreciate the ten minutes of your time and your support of others who want to love themselves and live in their Truth.

How to write me a review

Amazon US or UK: If you have an Amazon account that you've used in the last twelve months, you can type in "If you loved yourself—Eilat Aviram" and click on 'customer reviews' next to the stars under the book title.

Goodreads.com: Type in the name of this book. Underneath the book's cover image, hover over the stars until the desired number of stars is highlighted, then click on them to rate the book. A pop-up menu will appear above the stars. Click on the Write a review text. Enter your review on the following page, and click on Save to submit.

Barnes & Noble: Click on the 'Leave Your Review' button just under the Barnes & Noble heading.

BookBub (for US accounts): Click on the 'Review' button.

For those who love learning:

https://toughnickel.com/self-employment/How-to-Write-a-Book-Review-on-Amazon

https://www.dudleycourt-press.com/amazon-reviews-how-to-write-agood-book-review/

https://servenomaster.com/how-to-leave-an-amazon-video-review/

Acknowledgements

This started as 'I should probably thank some people' and ended up as a long love letter. And I couldn't even include everyone—but I tried.

Starting with my mother Adaya Rohloff-Aviram, because it started with you. Thank you for what you taught me—both with and without meaning to—about listening to my Truth and believing in and loving myself. I'm so proud of us for what we achieved together.

Shaul Freedman, my heart partner, father of my children, there are no words —and you don't like words anyway. I see you. Thank you for the depths of your support and dedication to us and your courage to let me fly.

Liran Freedman, my great teacher, you are wise and beautiful beyond measure. Your openness and constant loving support of all my ideas means so much to me. I love talking to you. I'm honored and overjoyed to be your mother.

Ellior Freedman, you are Love. Even your accidents. And you make me laugh and laugh. I learn from you every day and I'm so happy you came to me I can't even find the words.

My beloved father-in-law Nissim Chami, for being interested and asking me questions, loving me and being proud of me.

My editor Nicola Rijsdijk, what a journey we've had together. I'm really grateful for your partnering and support. Thank you for your excitement and for making this book more readable on so many levels.

Gill Strawberry Attwood, a shiny person, thank you for the beautiful front cover design and your PR magic. Your brilliant ideas come through so naturally you don't even notice what an impact you have.

Tarryn George, formatting together was total fun and you really held a beautiful space for me. I love the book design.

Christine Kloser, light-worker, author and teacher extraordinaire, it is a soul gratitude I extend to you. You blew my mind wide open to possibilities with your generous gift of the Transformational Author Experience. You have, quite literally, changed my life. Every author should have the privilege of engaging with you. Thank you beyond words for the work you do and for letting yourself shine.

To all the members of my tribe who have said and done just the right thing at the right time so that I could step further into my courage and expansion and Truth, my soul thanks you. I have felt supported by you and so proud to be connected with you. Eva Abrahams for always being there in the *most* important of ways and being genuinely excited about my journey. Molly Blank for that first conversation that birthed this idea and your editing. Zubeida Ahmed for encouraging me to be big and laughing with me. Rachel Wood, for you, and for That Talk by the lake. It grounded, cleared, relieved, inspired and gave me strength to go on. Dora Frasco for your huge vision, support, love and magic.And everyone in the community for being you and for showing up. Angelo Frasco for your challenge and insight and laughing at my woes in the best of ways. Melanie Meyer for helping me see what I can do. Elizabeth Nadler-Nir for your reading and affirmation. Rachael Sheriffs, for cheering me up and cheering me on. Meagan Hamman and Cherise Greenfield for kicking my butt into gear regarding indie publishing. My aunt Zahava Israeli for your tear-inducing unexpected show of love and support. My sisters Chemdat Aviram and Shlomit Cnaan for loving and accepting me like you do—and for your beauty and cleverness, of course.

IF YOU LOVED YOURSELF, WHAT WOULD YOU DO NOW?

To my beloved clients who've honored me with your stories, trust and love, you have no idea how much you teach and help me right back. I'd say something personal to you if I had space here. Your courage, honesty and beauty amazes and inspires me constantly. I feel like the luckiest person in the world to get to witness your journey and cheer you on.

To everyone I have not named here individually, and to all the light and energy workers out there—seen and unseen—I know that you know that I know that you know that I know what you have added to this endeavor. Because we are One. I thank you for looking at me with loving eyes and belief in my ability. I look at you the very same way. It has made this movement manifest.

Ok, that's enough. Now go love yourselves.

With love,

Eilat

www.eilataviram.com

Made in United States
Orlando, FL
13 June 2023